RUNNER'S WORLD.
RACE
EVERYTHING

How to Conquer Any Race at Any Distance in Any Environment and Have Fun Doing It

BART YASSO
with Erin Strout

RODALE.

RODALE *wellness*

Live happy. Be healthy. Get inspired.

Sign up today to get exclusive access to our authors, exclusive bonuses, and the most authoritative, useful, and cutting-edge information on health, wellness, fitness, and living your life to the fullest.
Visit us online at RodaleWellness.com
Join us at RodaleWellness.com/Join

© 2017 by Rodale Inc.

Rodale books may be purchased for business or promotional use or for special sales. For information, please e-mail BookMarketing@Rodale.com.

Runner's World is a registered trademark of Rodale Inc.

Printed in the United States of America
Rodale Inc. makes every effort to use acid-free ∞, recycled paper ♻.

Photos credits: AMCM/De Tienda/Mainguy, page 150; Atlanta Track Club/Paul Kim, page 46; Competitor Group, page 26; Crescent City Classic, page 44; Jesse Peters/Sports Backers, page 51; *Runner's World*/Jon Ivins, pages 129 & 130; *Runner's World*/Ryan Hulvat, pages 74, 75 & 76; and all others courtesy of Bart Yasso

Book design by Amy King

Library of Congress Cataloging-in-Publication Data is on file with the publisher.

ISBN 978-1-62336-982-8

Distributed to the trade by Macmillan
2 4 6 8 10 9 7 5 3 1 paperback

33614080434623

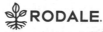

Follow us @RodaleBooks on 🐦 📘 📌 📷

We inspire health, healing, happiness, and love in the world.
Starting with you.

To the entire running community, I must thank you for keeping me motivated. Running with some of the kindest people on the planet has fueled me for the past 40 years.

I know I feel more like myself when I run, even if it's only a few miles—or at least I feel like the self I like best.

—Bart

CONTENTS

FOREWORD

In my 14 years as the editor in chief of *Runner's World,* I don't think I ever went to a race, big or small, where someone didn't ask me about Bart Yasso. Known for decades as "the mayor of running," and now *Runner's World's* chief running officer, Bart is the kind of guy you're proud to call your friend even if it doesn't make you feel at all unique. That's because Bart seems to know everyone, and everyone seems to know Bart. In airports, at race expos, at pasta dinners, and in porta-potty lines, they flock to him like long-lost relatives—and he usually remembers not only their names, but also their home-towns and marathon PRs.

Many years ago, I was looking at a stack of race photos in a common area of the *Runner's World* offices in Emmaus, Pennsylvania, for a story we were working on. Bart walked by and stopped to look through them with us. He paused on a shot of a pack of runners who had just crossed the starting line. I can't recall what race it was, but I remember that the photo was cropped at the runners' waists. Only their legs were visible. Bart pointed to a pair of men's gams and said, "I know that guy!" The runner's name has also vacated my memory all these years later, but Bart said it out loud. He might've added the guy's finishing time, too. I was too flabbergasted to notice, distracted by what I had just witnessed: Bart recognized one of his many running friends after *only seeing his legs.*

Bart has also been known to form bonds with runners he's never met, pilgrims who know the Legend of Bart even if they don't know the man himself. Joanna Golub, a *Runner's World* contributor who served as our nutrition editor for several years, once went hiking on a remote glacier in Alaska, hundreds of miles from civilization. At some point, she told her guide where she worked. "Oh, my God!" he exclaimed. "Do you know Bart Yasso?" Bart couldn't be on the glacier, but Joanna—who was just one degree of separation from the mayor—was the next best thing.

Bart's renown can be traced back, at least in part, to an unplanned and unintentional PR blitz that began as a slow boil in 1981. Bart, 25 at the time, decided he wanted to qualify for the Boston Marathon. He would need to run a 2:50 marathon—17 minutes faster than his PR—to do so. So he came up with a training routine to increase his speed. Once a week, in addition to his weekly workouts, he ran 800 meters on a track and then jogged 400 meters, eventually working up to 10 repetitions, or 7½ miles of running. It worked—he qualified for Boston by 1 second. So Bart continued to include this track workout in his training for other marathons, recording the results in his running log.

A few years later, he noticed an odd correlation between his marathon finishing times and the times in which he ran those 10 800-meter intervals. If he ran each interval around, say, 2 minutes and 40 seconds, his finishing time for the marathon was right around 2 hours and 40 minutes. If he ran them in 2:50—that is, 2 minutes and 50 seconds—that meant he was in shape to run a 2:50 marathon. This held true for 14 out of 15 marathons he ran since adopting this training regimen. Bart thought it was an interesting coincidence, but it wasn't until he casually mentioned it to Amby Burfoot, then the chief editor of *Runner's World,* that what are now known to runners around the world as Yasso 800s became a *thing.* Amby wrote a story about the workout and, in a surprise to Bart, even named it, explaining that when astronomers discover a new star, they get to name it whatever they want. So why shouldn't Bart get the credit?

If you Google "Yasso 800s" today, you will get more than 80,000 results. The workout, ideally done a few weeks before your goal race, has become a staple of marathon-training programs for all kinds of runners, from newbies to Olympic qualifiers. But even this cannot fully account for Bart's immense popularity. Yasso 800s may have earned him some coaching cred and name recognition, but he is beloved by legions of runners today not because of what he knows. It's because of what he's done and who he is.

Put simply, Bart has done more for runners and had more fun running than anyone I know. He recounted his many adventures and accomplishments—as well as the personal crises and challenges he has overcome along the way—in his 2008 memoir, *My Life on the Run*. If you're reading this, chances are you've read that book already. But if you haven't, you should. Bart has lived an amazing life.

For starters, he's traveled all over the world. His passport has been stamped with visas from Australia, New Zealand, Nepal, Peru, Kenya, Tanzania, India, and Egypt, among other far-flung nations. I guarantee that Bart met people in each of them that he would remember today if they ran into each other.

Of course, Bart has run races all over the world, too—more than he can even count. But it's not just his bucket list that makes Bart's running life—and this book—unique. It's his perspective. Bart can relate to all kinds of runners, from the front of the pack to the back, because he has *been* each of those runners in his lifetime. He won a marathon in his early years, and his PR is 2:40. He finished the Badwater Ultramarathon, widely regarded as one of the hardest footraces on earth. He's run the famed Comrades Marathon (a misnomer, since the course runs at least 56 miles, depending on whether it's an uphill or a downhill year) in South Africa. He once even ran neck and neck with 1972 Olympic marathon champion Frank Shorter in a race!

Despite all his accolades and achievements, Bart understands humility and remains authentically down-to-earth. He is personally acquainted with something all runners can relate to, regardless of how fast (or slow) they are: adversity. In 1990, Bart unknowingly contracted Lyme disease and, six years later, while climbing Mount Kilimanjaro in Africa, he suffered an attack of Bell's palsy that rendered the left side of his face and body temporarily paralyzed. These conditions have left Bart with joint pain and severe arthritis in his knee and hip. This has slowed him down, and at times it's hard for him to run more than a few easy miles. It hasn't stopped him from running—I don't think anything could—but it has given him a keen appreciation for how difficult, and yet therapeutic, running can be for so many people. Bart's PRs are behind him now, but he finds it just as fulfilling to participate in other ways, whether it's volunteering, coaching, race-directing, or helping out with the local running club.

When I started working at *Runner's World* in 2003, I must confess I didn't fully comprehend the power of Bart. I knew him as the guy who worked in the marketing department and rode his bike to work almost every day. At the time, *Runner's World* had a robust race-sponsorship program. We had partnerships with thousands of events across the country. This is why so many race bibs and swag bags have been emblazoned with the *Runner's World* logo over the years. Bart was our point of contact with all of the race directors in the program, and he spent nearly 200 days per year on the road, attending and running in races, sometimes doing some finish-line announcing or pasta-dinner speaking, always connecting with runners. This is how he got to know so many people, and, by extension, how he learned so much about the subculture that is road racing in America.

It quickly became clear to me that the amiable guy in the office down the hall was not only a font of insight and information, but also a vivid storyteller and a remarkable ambassador both for *Runner's World* and our sport. It also became clear that we should tap into Bart's vast knowledge and share it more widely with our readers. So in the January 2004 issue, which came out right around the time runners were planning the coming year's race calendar, we published a feature story entitled "Bart's Magical Marathon Tour." It was a roundup of Bart's favorite 26.2 milers, with quirky, plain-spoken explanations of what made each one great. It was a hit.

Since then, of course, Bart has written *My Life on the Run,* as well as dozens of articles and blog posts about running and racing. He has continued to travel the world, connecting with runners from big cities to small towns, from war zones to Amish country. He has also trained thousands of runners and inspired thousands more simply by being a positive, motivational example for people of all ages and abilities to emulate. I've seen it and heard about it firsthand more times than I can count.

A lot has changed since Bart started working at *Runner's World* in 1987. Race participation has exploded and the definition of "race" has evolved to include relays, mud runs, adventure races, and other unconventional events. Women have entered the sport in massive numbers, and they now outnumber men in some race distances, including the half marathon. And, of course, technology has transformed the way we track our running lives and connect with one another. Bart has celebrated and embraced it all. Despite the fact that the start of his running career preceded the digital age by a couple of decades, Bart took to social media instantly. After all, that's where the runners are, and now he can converse with tens of thousands of his followers at once from his office or his couch or whichever race he happens to be attending at the moment.

Perhaps it was inevitable, then, that Bart's digital skills would intersect with his itinerant job description to give us a new form of social interaction: the Bartie. It's no longer enough to merely meet Bart when one encounters him at a race or expo or pasta dinner. Now the interaction must be visually documented, and then shared as widely as possible. Sometimes Bart snaps the Barties himself, while other times his starstruck followers do. But the essential elements are the same either way: a camera or smartphone, Bart's face (or least some part of his head) in the foreground, and a group of happy runners (the more the better) in the background.

I took this Bartie during the 2016 *Runner's World* Half Marathon in Bethlehem, Pennsylvania. Bart was instrumental in founding the race—in the town where he grew up and still resides—and he designed the course himself. I don't know who the people behind us are, but Bart probably does. I keep it on my phone because it neatly represents our 14-year friendship and collaboration at *Runner's World*. It was the last race we ran together. Plus, I also live in Bethlehem, and the Bartie reminds me of how much work and energy we put into starting that race from scratch—and of how much fun we had putting it on every year. I know for sure that none of it would've happened if not for our CRO.

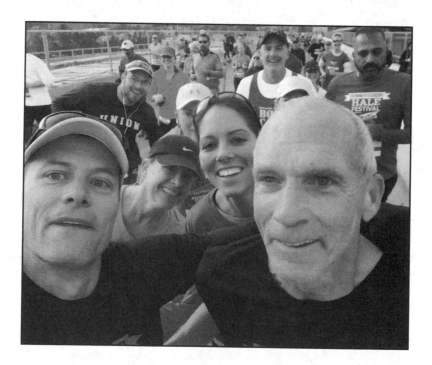

Bart knows as much as anyone I've ever met about races and racing. This book is a repository of all the knowledge and insider's expertise he has amassed over the decades. It's also a useful guide to running the world's very best races (from 5Ks through ultras, relays, triathlons, and unconventional events), and to running your very best in them (whatever "best" means to you, whether that's a PR or a first-time finish). It's packed with training plans, race-day tips, nutrition advice, and other indispensable wisdom. But unlike many guides and repositories, this book is also a joy to read. There are two reasons for this. First, Bart's steel-trap memory holds colorful details and hilarious anecdotes as easily as it stores names and faces. Second, Bart worked with the enormously talented Erin Strout, a *Runner's World* contributing editor, to get a lifetime of his stories and insights into these pages.

As you probably know, Bart will retire at the end of 2017. If you're lucky, you might see him at one of the races he recommends here. If you do, be sure to say hello—and follow it up with two simple words that only begin to account for all he has done, and continues to do, for the running community: Thanks, Bart.

And don't forget the Bartie.

—David Willey
July 2017

Chapter 1

The Many Reasons to Race

From fast times and personal records to adventures and camaraderie, the reasons we race are personal and diverse

It was the fall of 1977, and I was a 21-year-old who had wasted away my teen years on cigarettes, beer, and weed. I headed out for my first run in cutoff jeans cinched by a belt, a Budweiser T-shirt, and a pair of old Keds. I ran straight to a bar about a mile away. When I arrived, I celebrated by downing two beers—then I walked home.

It was an inauspicious start to a life forever changed by running. But it was a start nonetheless.

I had been inspired by my daily walks with my girlfriend's dog, Brandy, who showed unadulterated joy when she was liberated from her leash, free to romp and play. Those walks eventually morphed into runs by myself, gradually enjoying my own sense of freedom from the dark days I had fallen into. My older brother George—one of my six siblings—took notice of a kind of metamorphosis happening,

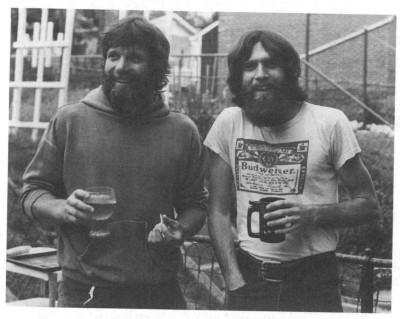

Bart (right) and his brother George enjoy some refreshments, probably after a run.

and as a father figure to me, he wanted to encourage this turning point in my life. By 1980 he goaded me into running a 10K with him in Moore Township, Pennsylvania, close to where we grew up in Fountain Hill. I had a giant, shaggy beard that covered most of my face; the other half was covered by my long, unkempt hair. It was decades before the advent of the selfie, but I looked like a running caveman. I was reluctant, and I had no idea what I was doing.

But most importantly, I showed up. And when the gun went off that morning, I shot out in a 5:20 first mile, naively going with a group of seasoned competitors in the lead pack. By mile two, I was predictably suffering a slow death and waning pace. By mile three, I wanted to vomit. George pulled away and never looked back. When I crossed the finish line in about 40 minutes, I had placed 40th out of 240 people. *Not bad,* I thought. Something inside was stirred.

When I headed back to my car that day, the windshield was

covered with fliers advertising other upcoming races in the area—
the 1980s equivalent of e-mail marketing. George was smart enough
to appeal to my competitive nature and challenged me to a rematch.
Three weeks later we were back on a 10K starting line, this time in
Easton, Pennsylvania, where I was struck by the challenge as well as
a new feeling of purpose. I held myself back for the first few miles,
then surged past George around mile five. By the time I reached that
finish line, I was aware on some subconscious level that my life
would never be the same. I was grateful. And I was, of course,
hooked. I couldn't wait to run my first marathon.

**Those first races left me hobbling around for days after-
ward.** In no way could I fathom that by trying a couple of 10K races,
I was embarking on a running career that would span more than
40 years. I didn't know that this sport would take me to events all
around the world, on all seven continents, running in at least 1,200
of the approximately 1,800 races I have attended. I've gone on to
contest distances from 1 mile to 146 miles, from Antarctica, South
Africa, India, and Rome, to Death Valley, Boston, New York, and
Chicago. Running has intimately connected me to a global community of active, health-conscious, and kind people. It's brought me
face-to-face with some of the most inspiring athletes on the planet.

What I've come to realize is that when the gun goes off, we all
follow the same course to the finish line, but each of us has taken a
different path to the starting line. Sometimes it's riddled with obstacles of every sort. Other times we are blessed with smooth sailing
from day one. But when you line up with hundreds or thousands of
others on race day, you will find hundreds or thousands of different
goals, expectations, and reasons for being there—all of them valid
and important. In my younger days, my sights were set on personal
records and maybe even a few wins. Now that I'm in my sixties, I
channel the same amount of passion toward merely finishing and
experiencing the joy of moving forward. I'm a little like Elvis—my

(continued on page 6)

Why Race?

The people on the sidelines shaking their heads, grumbling about the street closures, may never understand why so many of us rise with the roosters, put on our sneakers, and head to starting lines around the world every weekend. The easier choice is to sleep in, linger over the Sunday morning coffee, and read the newspaper.

Not all people who run choose to race, of course. But I've found that putting events on the calendar can lead to all sorts of good results—not only the kind that are measured by times and personal records, but those less-tangible, quality-of-life ways, too.

Here are my top reasons runners should consider racing.

1. **Accountability.** Running every day is an accomplishment. Heck, running just a few times a week is an achievement, too. But registering for a race and forking over some hard-earned dollars gives your running increased importance and priority. Now you're account-able because you have to be prepared to run to the best of your ability on a specified date. That doesn't necessarily mean that you're going to run your fastest, but it does mean you have committed to train as well as you can to cover the distance. Sometimes you just need to give yourself a deadline and a race will inevitably jump-start your routine.

2. **Fitness tests.** Often, races are just measuring sticks—opportunities to gauge where our fitness is and where it needs to improve. It's easier to give yourself an honest check when you've pinned a race bib to your shirt and lined up with other people. You're not there to compare yourself with everybody else, but the presence of those around you can bring more out of you than just another time trial by yourself. This isn't a pass/fail test—it's just a way to find out what you need to work on next.

3. **A change of scenery.** Every runner gets stuck in a rut once

in a while, when training feels forced and the drudgery of the routine starts to wear us down. To me that is the perfect time to scan the Internet for events that offer some sort of new challenge or are in a place you've wanted to visit, but never had reason to go. You can find races in every corner of the world if you look hard enough. Finding one that stokes new inspiration or excitement can get you back on track.

4. **Camaraderie.** I say it over and over again, but truly the greatest gift that running has given me is this global community of like-minded people, most of whom I've met because of all the races I attend. If you train mostly on your own and you are looking for buddies, the first place to find them is at a race. You can strike up a conversation with just about anybody and it's not even awkward. There's a genuine "we're all in this together" mentality among runners on a starting line.

5. **Inspiration from the top.** One of the most unique parts about our sport is that anybody of any age or skill level can run the same race as the professional athletes. Those poor saps who take to the league basketball team will never play in the same game or on the same court as Steph Curry, but we runners line up behind Shalane Flanagan, Desiree Linden, and Meb Keflezighi all the time. They may finish hours ahead of us, but we're following in their footsteps every step of the way. And that's pretty cool.

6. **Inspiration from everywhere else, too.** I leave races in awe of the accomplishments of so many different kinds of people. There are the older runners still crushing their goals. Then we see the newer people, some of them trying to lose a few pounds or just run farther than they ever have before. People run while fighting cancer and other illnesses—their strength and determination is beyond

(continued)

Why Race? *(cont.)*

admirable. If you're looking for motivation, it's everywhere. If you leave a race without being touched by it, make sure you still have a heart.

7. **Be better than before.** Most of us aren't there to win any prize money, though if that is your goal, more power to you and good luck! Races are the obvious place to go to be our best, to try to run faster than we ever have before. It's you against the clock, you against a former version of yourself. A race can be a big turning point, a confidence booster, and an indication that you have more ability than you thought possible. Dreams come true at races. Just stand at a finish line for 15 minutes and watch the reactions of everybody reaching new heights.

8. **Lend encouragement.** Even on the days that don't go our way, these events are also a setting where we can help others achieve their goals. If you're not feeling 100 percent, don't hit snooze. Wake up, get yourself to the starting line, and help somebody else. Pace a friend or merely cheer on the people around you. You'll be surprised how fulfilling it can be to spur somebody else on to her own greatness.

9. **Support a good cause.** So many events now donate proceeds to charities. Even if you're not looking to blaze a new personal record, you can still sign up to run and know that your money is doing some good in the community.

10. **Long-run support.** If you're at that point of marathon training when the long runs are getting really long, signing up for a race as part of that day's training can help the miles fly

speed (and a lot of my hair!) has left the building, but my spirit soars on.

I'm now untied from my race clock, happy to let it tick away while I take my time to meet new people and look at the scenery. That wasn't always the case, though. My watch determined the success or failure of decades' worth of running, until time was no longer worth chasing.

by. If you have a 20 miler on your plate, make a 10K part of it by running some of the miles beforehand and some afterward. The race portion of the long run can serve as a tempo or as the pace-work portion of the run. You'll have instant running buddies, water stops, and even restrooms readily available, should you need any of those amenities. And you'll probably get a medal or a T-shirt for your efforts, which never happens after your typical Sunday morning grind.

11. **Fun.** Right. Did I forget to mention that running is supposed to be fun? Race events try to make it that way. Bands, food, festival-like finish line areas—it's a celebration of running. You can't help but get caught up in the atmosphere and smile. And smiling is a per-fectly legal performance enhancer—we should all do it more often.

12. **Get out of your comfort zone.** Registering for a race in which you've set a big, scary goal or one that's farther than you've ever gone before is uncomfortable. The butterflies and anxiety-ridden prerace dreams confirm that. But there's no better feeling than facing that kind of fear, staring it down, and learning you're more capable than you realized. These kinds of racing moments transfer to every other aspect of our lives, somehow making us realize we can excel in our careers, relationships, and other areas we hope to improve. We open doors to all sorts of possibilities with each finish line we cross.

My first bout of Lyme disease was in 1990, just after I finished the Lake Waramaug 50 miler in Connecticut. In a short span of time I went from running 50 miles in 6 hours and 11 minutes to struggling to cover 1 mile. I was misdiagnosed and went untreated for a long time; after I was put on the appropriate antibiotics, it took a few months to resume my running routine. I came back strong as a 43-year-old, with a 2:42 at the California International Marathon.

My health remained stable until 1997, and this time Lyme almost cost me my life. A tick bite that I probably sustained on the trails in Pennsylvania caused severe illness during a trip to East Africa, but I fought back again through a long hiatus to win the Smoky Mountain Marathon. A third bout of the disease awaited me in 2002, and when I left the hospital, I never regained my prior fitness level.

I am humbled to run a few miles a week now, aware and respectful of what my body can muster. The people I meet in the running community inspire me to keep going—I've slowed down tremendously, but my connection with the sport has only strengthened.

In this book we'll explore not only some of the reasons to consider races of many distances, but how to train for them, which ones I've enjoyed most, and what to expect at the most unique and prestigious events I've run. I'll give you a taste of my personal experiences and why each of these races has become a special part of my running story. From Comrades, my favorite race of all time, to the Monument Avenue 10K in Richmond, Virginia, to the *Runner's World* Half Marathon in my own backyard of Bethlehem, Pennsylvania, I've learned how to best prepare for varying terrain, large crowds, and all kinds of weather conditions, as well as how to adjust physically and emotionally to the many unforeseen circumstances that arise when getting ready to tackle a big goal.

But perhaps the greatest lesson you will glean from me is to never limit where your running can take you. Indeed, it's taken me almost everywhere—and if that can happen to me, it can happen to anyone. Run a marathon in all 50 states or on all 7 continents. Or choose just one 10K. Tackle the summer 5K series in your hometown. Dare to finish an ultramarathon. Or gather up a team and hit the relay circuit. The running world has so much to offer to all ages and abilities, the hardest part is figuring out which path to choose.

Racing defines our running, provides start dates and end dates, measures our progress, and gives reasons to celebrate. It offers a chance to learn how to prepare and how to execute. The most meaningful part of racing for me has been the opportunity to experience new cultures and see parts of the world I'd otherwise miss.

My life has been molded and framed by the weekends spent traveling to starting lines all around the world. It's been expanded by adventures that have happened on the way to all those finish lines. I wish the same for every runner, and I believe that no matter what your aspirations, it is racing that brings a sense of structure, camaraderie, motivation, and achievement to our running.

When I travel to events as *Runner's World*'s chief running officer, my hope is always to inspire others the way that George encouraged me so many years ago. Whatever your reason, you, too, can race everything.

Chapter 2

Bart's Training Principles

The fundamentals of preparing for any distance include workouts, mileage, and how to progress safely

Racing, of course, takes preparation no matter what your ability level or objectives. When I first became interested in performance goals, I bought *The Complete Book of Running* by Jim Fixx. It was my running Bible, my go-to manual for every training-related question I had, and it was fortuitous that it came out when it did—during what many called the first "running boom." As I researched more about the sport, I always seemed to gravitate back to that book, like many runners of the '80s. It was what popularized running during that era. Who could forget that cover, with those muscular running legs, angled in perfect form, and those bright red shorts?

But as my racing experiences began to expand, so did my need for more personalized advice. That's when I met Budd Coates, who owned a personal best of 2:13 in the marathon and had qualified for the Olympic Trials four times. He was the director of fitness and health at Rodale Inc., the company based in Emmaus, Pennsylvania, that owns *Runner's World*. Amid hill workouts and track sessions, Budd taught me how to lead a runner's lifestyle. He was a master at his craft, and I wanted to emulate that. I wanted to do as he did. He told me that merely logging mileage would never make me faster—I had to also pay attention to nutrition, the amount of sleep I was getting, strength training, and flexibility, among other things. I learned from him that all the decisions I made outside of running had a true impact on my success as a runner. Budd and Amby Burfoot, former editor in chief of *Runner's World* and 1968 Boston Marathon champion, have always been instrumental in my running career.

When I was hired by *Runner's World* as the race and event coordinator in 1987, my job was to forge relationships on behalf of the magazine with race directors across the country. As I traveled to more events and attended countless expos, it was also my responsibility to connect with as many runners as possible. Somewhere along the line, those conversations turned to questions about training and racing (or shoes or nutrition or . . . you name it, I've discussed it with more than one runner!). And the more conversations I had, the more runners began to view me as an expert—a running coach to the masses. Back at home, my local group, the Lehigh Valley Road Runners, leaned on me to come up with workouts and man the watch at practices.

Through trial, error, and a lot of observation, I came to realize that successful training is a highly individualized endeavor. We know that what works for one runner may not work for another. We all come to running with different goals, DNA, physiological attributes, and levels of motivation. A training plan not only has to take into account all of this, but your other life circumstances—like jobs, family commitments, and anything else that requires your attention. We all have a finite amount of time and energy, so it's up to each of us to decide how much of it can be spent on running.

Training can be as simple or as complicated as we want it to be, depending on our experience and our racing goals. Add in strength training, core work, flexibility, and cross-training, and the sky's the limit for how many elements can be part of a plan. A few basic training principles, however, stand the test of time for nearly every runner—implementing them in a manner that meets your individual needs is critical.

Here are the key areas I consider when creating a plan for a race of any distance, influenced by my own running throughout the decades, the feedback I hear from runners of all abilities, and those whom I've been fortunate to learn from, like Budd and Amby.

MILEAGE

Running is the only activity that will make you a better runner. That's a basic concept, right? Building up your mileage, however, isn't as easy as it might seem. If you're doing it correctly, you'll gradually increase the volume of miles you run per week over time. If you fall into the "terrible toos" by doing too much, too soon, too often, you risk injury, illness, and burnout. Piling on miles before you're ready is too difficult to sustain for the long haul and is crying out for trouble.

Mileage comes in various forms, but for me the bulk of it has always been done at an easy pace several days per week. It's important to keep easy days at a pace that is comfortable—you shouldn't have any problem talking with your friends if you're doing it right. Even the world's best runners take their easy-day pace seriously because if they overdo the intensity on those runs, they will not be able to complete their speed workouts as fast as they should. The same applies to the rest of us—the easy mileage is what builds our aerobic system and strengthens our muscles.

Increasing your mileage is important as you begin to see

improvements, but you have to do it safely. An old rule of thumb is to take your baseline mileage—what you know you can complete each week comfortably—and add no more than 10 percent to that in a week. However, it's wise to sometimes keep your mileage the same for 2 consecutive weeks to make sure you're adapting to the increased load without hurting yourself. You can add miles to a weekly total by increasing the number of days per week that you run or by extending the duration of a few of your easy runs.

Mileage is also dependent on the race distance you're targeting. We'll get into that in more detail in the following chapters. The longer the distance, the more miles you will need to run. The shorter the distance, the more you will focus on the quality of your miles— meaning you'll likely have less overall mileage, but you'll probably be running more of those miles at a faster pace to prepare for a shorter, quicker race. If your goal is merely to finish a race and you're not worried about your time, your mileage can be less.

LONG RUNS

The long run is a weekend ritual for many of us, along with the customary coffee and brunch gathering afterward. Going long once a week helps improve our endurance and strength and can include practicing specific paces you might use in your goal race. The distance of the long run is dependent on what race you're training for and your experience level. But no matter if you're targeting a 5K or an ultramarathon, those long runs are a critical part of the plan.

Some runners measure their long runs in minutes instead of miles because they're more concerned about practicing the time on their feet than covering the exact number of miles that might be prescribed by a different strategy—this is a good way to start implementing long runs if you're new to running or if you're training for an ultra distance (anything longer than 26.2 miles). But I've learned that this method, though useful for many, does not work for me. I am more confident on race day if I know that I've successfully covered a 20-mile training run as opposed to a 3-hour run. I really enjoy a long run that feels comfortable, often at a pace a minute per mile slower than what I hope to keep during the race—we call this LSD in the business, which stands for "long, slow distance."

Some runners like to break up a few of their long runs with pace work, which is a good idea if you've moved past the beginner phase. You can come up with a lot of variations to include some speed in a long run. For those training for a marathon, for example, maybe a 16-mile run will include 4 miles easy, 4 miles at goal marathon pace, and then repeat that sequence. If you're training for a shorter distance, a good way to incorporate a little bit of speed into a long run might be a progression—start out slow and gradually speed up until the last mile or two is your race pace.

WORKOUTS

Workouts usually refer to those sessions we do once or twice a week that require speed of some kind. They can occur on a track, road, hill, or trail. The great thing about workouts is that there are so many kinds of them, you'll never get bored. There are probably just as many good reasons to do workouts as varieties you can choose from. It's speed sessions that help us become fitter and faster. They tax a different system than all those easy miles, teach us how to pace ourselves, and to a certain extent can also allow us to learn how to cope with being uncomfortable. And they serve as just one more way to improve performance. When you learn how to run faster at shorter intervals, eventually your easy pace and race pace improve, too. Many studies also show that interval training is essential to weight loss, if shedding a few pounds is a goal of yours.

HILLS: One of my favorite workouts is hill repeats. We have a lot of hills where I live in eastern Pennsylvania, and I enjoy the combination of running hilly courses on my long runs and then doing some hill repeats during the week. It's nearly impossible to get up a hill using bad running form—when you're powering an ascent you naturally lift your knees higher and swing your arms forward, which also forces a speedier cadence and a better stride. Long hills, short hills, steep hills, and gradual hills all build desirable muscle strength in different ways, and all can be used to prepare for a variety of terrains and race distances.

Some races, like the Boston Marathon, demand that runners also practice downhill running to strengthen the quads, which take a beating over the first half of the course. Downhill workouts, which I'll talk about more in the following chapters, teach you how to avoid leaning back, overstriding, and braking—all of which are bad form. You want to practice leaning slightly forward from the ankles and letting gravity do the work. I like to picture the form of a ski jumper to give myself a visual cue for how I should approach a downhill.

My mantra for going uphill or downhill is simple: nose over toes. If your nose isn't over your toes, you're probably overstriding.

STRIDES: Strides are an easy way to sneak in a little bit of speedwork a few times a week. They're also a good way for beginners to ease into a little bit of faster running without getting wrapped up in a track workout. Strides are 15 to 20 seconds of running at about 85 to 90 percent effort (fast, but not all-out), with full recovery in between—doing four to six of them after a short, easy run two or three times a week wakes up those fast-twitch muscles and gets your legs turning over faster. They're best done on a flat surface, such as a parking lot or a grassy field.

FARTLEKS: An oldie but a goodie. For the uninitiated, a fartlek isn't some kind of middle-school cafeteria humor—it's the Swedish word for "speed play." You don't need any specific kind of terrain to do a fartlek run—it works just the same on a road, trail, track, or even a treadmill. All you have to do is implement intervals of hard running, followed by easy running. For example, after an easy 1 or 2 miles, spend the next 20 minutes running 1 minute "on"/1 minute "off" ("on" is harder and faster effort and "off" is easy pace). After implementing fartleks into your routine, you will gradually build your aerobic capacity until you're able to maintain a faster pace for a longer period of time with less effort.

TRACK WORKOUTS: The track can be an intimidating or anxiety-ridden place for some runners. For many, it brings back terrible flashbacks of the timed mile in gym class or visions of the world's fastest athletes hunched over in agony at the finish line. While speed sessions at the track can be demanding, they also should be run according to your ability level, which should ease a little bit of the fear. Track workouts are a good way to learn and practice precise pacing—it's an exactly measured 400-meter oval on a flat surface, which makes everything easier. My favorite track workouts, of course, are Yasso 800s (see page 18), but the basic premise of a track workout is similar to a fartlek: hard, fast bouts of running, followed by intervals of recovery, either walking or jogging. The intervals and paces are dependent on what you're training for, your experience level, and your goals. An easy beginner workout is running the straightaways at a harder effort, then jogging the curves. You can progress to more specific workouts of varying intervals from there.

TEMPO RUNS: The tempo pace is what runners like to call "comfortably hard," which sounds like an oxymoron. How can something hard feel comfortable? Truth be told, tempo pace doesn't really feel comfortable—it's a speed that isn't easy, but that you can sustain over longer distances; for most people, a good measurement is what they can sustain at a hard effort for 1 hour. It's an important workout, especially for half marathons and marathons. Implementing a tempo run into your weekly routine teaches your body to use

A Word about Yasso 800s

Perhaps what I've become most famous for in the running community is a little workout that became known as Yasso 800s.

Back in 1981 my goal was to run a 2:50 marathon so I could qualify for Boston. I kept meticulous training logs back then, though it wasn't until about 3 years later, when I read some of my training cycles, that I noticed a trend in my speed workouts. It seemed that the average time it took me to run 10 x 800 meters always corresponded to my marathon finish times. So if I could run 10 x 800 meters with each 800-meter interval in 2 minutes and 40 seconds with a 400-meter recovery jog in between,

my marathon time would be right around 2:40. I'd do this several times in my marathon buildup.

Believe me when I say that I didn't think I had cracked some miraculous marathon running code. I had simply found a system that worked for me. It wasn't until 1993 that I shared it with Amby Burfoot, who was the editor of *Runner's World* at the time. We were rooming together at the Portland Marathon and I was training for the Marine Corps Marathon. He asked what my goal was that year and I said I knew I was going to run a 2:47. Then I explained how I knew this precise goal to be true, laying out the details of my 800s workout

lactate more effectively, delaying the point that your legs begin to fatigue—or pushing your lactate threshold a little farther.

There are many forms of tempo runs, but the easiest way to get started is to first find your pace. You don't have to enter a lab and give away your blood to find it, either. Take a recent 5K or 10K race result and add 10 to 20 seconds to your average pace per mile. Or, if you're using perceived effort, the difficulty level should be around 8 on a scale of 10, with 10 being most difficult. A solid workout: 15 to to him. Amby's curiosity was piqued.

While nobody to this day can explain why this accidental method works for so many people, after some experimentation and number crunching, Amby was so convinced of its authenticity that he put the workout in the October 1994 issue of the magazine. What did he call them? Much to my surprise at the time, he dubbed them Yasso 800s.

When you have a workout named after you, you get a lot of what I will graciously call "feedback." I tend to hear a lot of gratitude from those who've had success with it, but I also hear from many who have tried it without that kind of luck. Every day on social media I see somebody cursing my name, and I'm okay with that. Curse away. Yasso 800s don't account for the conditions of every marathon. Will it be hilly? Hot? Windy? The Yasso 800 workout doesn't know. But the runner does and should adjust their expectations accordingly.

What the Yasso 800 workout will gauge well is your fitness. If you do 10 x 800 meters, with a 400-meter recovery jog in between each one, about 5 weeks before your marathon at a pace that targets your goal, and you feel good doing it, my guess is that you are in for a great race.

20 minutes easy, 20 minutes at threshold pace, then 15 minutes of cooldown.

More-experienced runners can spend more time at threshold pace during a workout—and probably should in order to get the maximum benefits and results. Some half marathoners can incorporate up to 8 miles of a long run at tempo pace, while marathoners might work up to 13 miles at threshold. You can also try two sets of 30 minutes at half-marathon pace or 1 hour at marathon pace.

REST AND RECOVERY

It's among the most overlooked and poorly executed parts of training—getting enough rest and recovery. I strongly believe in the critical part that rest plays in performance. After you've put in all the training, the body needs time to adapt to the new demands you've put on it. Many coaches call it "stress, then rest." When your body is allowed to recover adequately, it repairs the damage you've inflicted on your muscles, regenerates your immune and endocrine systems, and begins to reap the fitness gains you're working toward. The body bounces back with proper recovery and prepares itself for more work.

Runners who don't get adequate recovery are usually the ones who are battling the most injuries and illnesses. They are mentally burned out, and their workouts begin to crumble. Proper recovery comes in many forms. During a heavy training period, recovery includes getting enough sleep each night, making sure you're eating nourishing and nutritious food (and enough of it), and staying hydrated. I am a proponent of taking at least one day off from running each week. Sometimes I cross-train on the bike, on the elliptical, or in the pool on those off days, but you can also just rest completely while you're training for a race. If you choose to cross-train, I suggest keeping the intensity low and allowing yourself to just reap the benefits of gentle movement and blood circulation without impact—some people call this "active recovery."

Over time you will learn to listen to the signals your body is sending. There's a difference between feeling the general fatigue of training, which is natural and nothing to worry about, versus training too hard. If you dig yourself into a hole of overtraining, it's difficult to get back out. A few signs that could indicate you should take an extra rest day include:

- ➤ An elevated resting heart rate

- ➤ Loss of appetite

- ➤ Inability to sleep well, despite feeling tired

- ➤ Being overly grumpy or emotional for no reason

- ➤ Trudging through workouts that aren't going well

The most successful runners are those who are able to train consistently over many years. The only way to do that is to make sure you're taking planned breaks—as opposed to the forced variety due to injuries and illness. I advocate that runners take a break twice a year for 10 days to 2 weeks each. Taking time off after a big goal race will allow your body to recover from the effort and also allow your mind to disengage for a little while. It's as much a physical need as it is a psychological one—we want to enjoy running for many years, but that's unlikely to happen if you overdo it. If life is unexpectedly busy due to work or family commitments, it's also a good time to ease off on training.

CROSS-TRAINING

I enjoy cross-training more than many other runners do, and I think it's good to incorporate some of it into a training schedule. The key is to not overdo it. You're obviously training to run a race, so spending too much time on an elliptical isn't going to help you achieve your goals. However, spending 30 minutes or an hour doing some sort of nonimpact activity on a rest day can help you torch a few more calories and get some blood circulating through your recovering muscles.

A lot of people come to me for cross-training advice, and the one thing I tell them is that you don't want to wait until you're injured

Becoming a Multisport Athlete

I haven't always just focused on running during my career. My love for bicycling has led me on some of the most grand adventures of my life, including riding across the country twice.

It was in the mid-1980s that I discovered duathlons—races that combine bicycling and running. I found that I enjoyed the diversity of the sport and lined up for about 20 of them in 1986. Then in 1987 I won the US Biathlon Association Long Course Championship—a 6-mile run, a 45-mile bike ride, and another 6-mile run. Breaking the tape there was a fantastic memory, and *Sports Illustrated* even did a story about me after that happened, which was quite an honor.

The first time I biked across the country, I flew from Lehigh Valley Airport out to Seattle to begin my journey all the way back to Asbury Park, New Jersey. I went with no crew on a self-support trek, which took me 20 days. I loved that trip so much, I did it again 2 years later.

While I've always loved running the most, I think that trying other sports and activities has prolonged my ability to remain active. Not only has it helped me stay fit and healthy, but also mentally engaged. And I wouldn't trade the stories and the people I met along the way during those cross-country journeys for anything. Few days go by when I don't think about those 3,000-mile solo trips—just me and my bike and this diverse, beautiful country.

to cross-train. I do it to avoid injuries—if I ran 7 days a week at this point, I'd get hurt. But I can keep my fitness level up if I ride the bike or hop on the elliptical in addition to running. Many elite runners who don't want to run twice a day substitute a run with some sort of other activity, such as swimming, to lessen the chances of getting hurt while still getting the aerobic benefits that a run would provide.

The best kind of cross-training activities are the ones that you enjoy and you'll look forward to doing. Deep-water running, riding a bike, going for a hike, or swimming laps are all beneficial. The key is to be consistent. I recommend cross-training about two times per week—and maybe even more during breaks from running.

FLEXIBILITY, CORE, AND STRENGTH

We call the other recommended activities that supplement training "ancillary," but I'd argue that they're a necessary component of race preparation. Flexibility, core, and a little bit of general strength training can help keep you injury-free, and they also contribute to better overall running performance.

I go to the gym two times per week, and I think of two words when I go there: *strength* and *flexibility*. Every workout I do has some combination of the two. I especially believe that a strong core is critical—it helps you maintain your running posture even when you're tired, and I've found it also helps my breathing. When I'm beginning to fade and fatigue, I'm still able to sustain my pace because of the work I do at the gym.

I also believe that focusing on my flexibility and general strength has allowed me to stay healthy. I've had very few injuries over the years beyond those that are a result of my Lyme disease. I don't focus too much on lifting heavy weights, but I'll do higher repeats with lighter weights to maintain my strength.

It's good to find a routine that works for you. There are a lot of options to fit these activities into your schedule in a way you enjoy. Yoga is a really good supplement to running, or you can find several body-weight workouts that don't take much time and can be done at home. Routines that aid strengthening all the little muscles and ligaments that support your running and work your balance are helpful. Planks, lunges, squats—they all go a long way toward better running and longevity in the sport, which I will cover more extensively in Chapter 10.

Chapter 3

Training for and Racing 5Ks

Choosing and preparing for a 5K, race strategies, and key workouts

When I started running competitively in the early 1980s, the 5K distance wasn't as prevalent as it is today—it was the 10K that drew most road racers back then. As running became more popular not just as a sport, but as a fitness activity, the 3.1-mile race started dominating the scene. Now you can find multiple 5Ks in nearly every community, any time of the year, throughout the country. In fact, according to Running USA statistics, the 5K is the most popular distance in the United States—it typically accounts for about 45 percent of all runners who complete races each year.

Why do runners flock to the 5K? For beginners, it's an approachable distance to train for because it's just long enough to feel like an accomplishment and short enough not to be too intimidating. The 5K is also accessible—with so many to choose from (more than 16,000 of them annually), you don't need to travel far or plan ahead

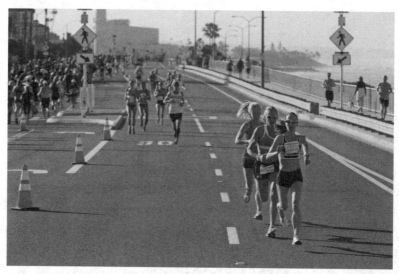

The Carlsbad 5000, which runs along the Pacific Ocean in Southern California, is one of Bart's longtime favorite races.

to race one. If you're feeling fit and ready, there's usually a 3.1-mile race somewhere close by to jump into. If it doesn't go well? Sign up for another one next weekend—unlike a marathon, you don't have to wait several months to take another stab at it. And for the more experienced runners who are trying to get faster, the 5K is the ultimate test of speed and strength, all in one shot.

One of my earliest memories of the 5K distance is lining up at a local race near Bethlehem with Budd Coates and Mark Will-Weber, a senior editor at *Runner's World* who was another accomplished runner like Budd and had a list of personal best times much more impressive than my own. I don't so much remember what happened during that race, other than putting myself in the hurt zone and experiencing some fierce lung burn, but I do remember receiving a lot of accolades and recognition from the race director while we were lining up on the start line. I had recently finished Badwater—which was then a 146-mile ultramarathon (it's now a mere 135 miles) through Death Valley to Mount Whitney, dubbed the "World's Toughest Footrace"—and upon returning home to the Lehigh Valley,

I was receiving a startling amount of recognition for that feat. In fact, my new nickname became Badwater Bart. There I was, ready to run this 5K, knowing that Mark and Budd were the real contenders in the field, and the only person the director introduced before the gun went off was me. I thought, *I could get used to this 5K business.*

Of course that race was not my most notorious 5K by a long stretch. In 1997 I lined up au naturel for the Bare Buns Fun Run at Kaniksu Ranch, a family nudist resort in Washington State. I had been asked to attend the in-the-buff event and be the guest speaker at the prerace pasta dinner. So I stood without a stitch of clothing on, before a room full of runners, and gave my usual motivational pep talk. This time I didn't have the option to imagine my audience naked if I got nervous because they were already sans clothing. I wasn't sure what other coping mechanisms were recommended under these circumstances.

Alas, I remained disrobed for the entirety of the weekend, including the 5K the next morning, where I affixed my race bib to my arm with a piece of yarn. It felt odd—though entirely liberating and surprisingly comfortable—to race naked. Even the aid station volunteers, who donned orange vests, wore no pants. The only body parts that were covered for most of the runners were our feet—running shoes were, thankfully, allowed for those of us competing in the textile-free division, which was nearly everybody.

It wasn't easy to stay focused, but my competitive side surfaced toward the end of the race, when another runner caught me, instigating a full-fledged sprint toward the finish line. I won the masters division and ironically collected a finisher's T-shirt that said, "I ran nude at the Bare Buns Fun Run."

I have yet to run any other 5Ks in the flesh, but the point is that you can find a 5K to fit any need. If you want to support a charity, race a competitive field, go for a personal record, or try something wacky (Donut Dash, anybody?), chances are an event of the 3.1-mile distance has been created to fulfill your every racing desire.

As for the Bare Buns Fun Run, it now bills itself as the

second-oldest race in the region behind Bloomsday, the 12K in Spokane, Washington, that attracts more than 42,000 participants in May. At the Bare Buns, you can expect a smaller crowd of about 300 people, but you'll be exposed to so much more of them.

BART'S FAVORITE 5K: THE CARLSBAD 5000

One of my all-time favorite 3.1-mile races is in Carlsbad, California—it's the world-renowned Carlsbad 5000, where all runners get the chance to line up and compete head-to-head with their own age groups, in separate men's and women's heats. The day, usually in late March or early April, turns into a seaside festival of 5K races, and the atmosphere is second to none.

Usually when you go to an event with family or friends, you don't get to watch each other race. At Carlsbad, you have a better shot at cheering one another on. The day begins with the masters men's heat, followed by masters women a little more than an hour later. Then men and women ages 29 and under get their chance, followed by the 30 to 39 group about 90 minutes after that. After the wheelchair race finishes, it's time to watch the elite races. They are really exciting to spectate because Carlsbad draws many of the fastest 5K runners in the world—16 world records and 8 American records were set in the first 31 editions of the event.

In the early years, the men's professional race was contested by Steve Scott, who once held the American mile record three different times, plus earned a 1983 world championships silver medal in the 1500 meters. Beginning at the inaugural race in 1986, Steve won Carlsbad three consecutive times. Later, I got to witness Sammy Kipketer, of Kenya, race Carlsbad, which he won 3 years in a row as well. In 2000 and 2001, he dipped below 13 minutes, finishing in 12:59.5 and 12:59.6, which were then course records (the course has since changed for the elite races). Meseret Defar, from Ethiopia, ran the fastest women's time on the original course in 2006 with a 14:46.

But the pro runners aren't the only ones who can push themselves on a course like Carlsbad. For the recreational runners, it's a good place to set a personal record, not only because of the mostly flat terrain, but because it's so spectator friendly that you can't help but absorb the electricity of the crowd. I've raced it several times, mostly in the late 1990s and early 2000s. In my division—the men's 40 and older—you'd see these guys going through the first mile in 5:10 at 69 years old. I was continually blown away by how talented the fields could be, though the concept and the venue are welcoming to all ability levels. In 2000, I did a 17-mile run prior to the start because I was training for a marathon at the time, and I still clocked a 17:18 in the race. That was a fun way to do a long run and a good way to add a fast-finish element to it, which you could do in conjunction with any 5K race.

Racing Tips for the Carlsbad 5000

The 3.1-mile course is mostly flat, with ever-so-slight undulations throughout, ending on a bit of a downhill to the finish line. Runners spend most of the race next to the Pacific Ocean, so there can be a little bit of a breeze, but usually it's more refreshing than bothersome.

➤ Parking in Carlsbad can be tricky, so leave yourself plenty of time to find a space and continue on with your prerace routine.

➤ The course has two notable turnaround points that slow most people down momentarily. Think about how you'll negotiate those turns. Will you swing wide? Or cut in close and make them sharp? Consider practicing a few turns during your training, if you're going for a new personal best. Set up a couple of cones in a parking lot, for example, and practice approaching them at full speed so you are mentally prepared to run them on race day.

➤ As the day progresses, the best spectating spots near the finish get taken quickly. If you want to see friends race or the elites compete, have a plan ready to nab a good spot after you've finished your race.

➤ Like any big race, make sure you're lining up at the appropriate spot for your predicted pace. If you get stuck behind a lot of people who are going much slower than you, you'll have a hard time getting past them in the first half mile. Conversely, if you're lining up with people who are planning a much faster pace than you, you might blow your race strategy.

➤ That said, the first mile can be incredibly quick. Make sure you're running your own race and not getting caught up in the excitement and adrenaline of the people around you. If you mess up the first mile of a 5K, the rest is going to get ugly. You will want to waste no time getting on your goal pace, but feel controlled enough that you don't blow it so early in the race.

TRAINING FOR A 5K

The 5K demands a unique mixture of aerobic capacity and speed, so training for this distance is never boring—you can tap into multiple physiological systems and log a decent number of miles, too, though the point is to increase the quality of the runs over the quantity. Spending some time preparing for the 5K can naturally lead to faster paces all around, especially for those who tend to focus more on mileage than quality speed sessions. Basically, if you want to get faster at longer distances, you have to get faster at shorter distances first. Makes sense, right?

For those who are newer to running and targeting a 5K as a first race, there are plenty of benefits to training for this distance as well. It will naturally improve endurance and strength. Research shows that interval training, which is added in after adequate base mileage has been mastered, can torch calories quicker, leading to weight loss. That's good news if you're hoping to shed a few pounds as you get fitter.

Here are some sample training plans for the 5K distance. Remember that not all runners respond to training in the same way,

Bart's Favorite 5K Workout

My favorite track workout when I was training for 3.1-mile races was 20 x 400 meters with a 200-meter recovery jog in between them. We used to do these by feel rather than by our specific 5K goal pace. *Note: This workout is not for new runners.*

Back then we didn't have watches that kept track of the splits for us. Have you ever tried to count 20 intervals while you're in a hypoxic state? Instead, we'd line up 20 little rocks on the start line and kick one away every time we were done with a repeat. You'd see the number of pebbles decreasing, but you'd fear that your buddies were putting them back when you weren't looking, forcing you to unknowingly complete more intervals than planned. Not nice.

Needless to say, I love technology now. Nobody can mess with your workout anymore.

But back to the task at hand. Although most runners like to hit exact times during workouts, you don't always need to be so precise. Learning your perceived exertion has many benefits, including the fact that you may actually be limiting your potential by targeting a specific pace you want to hit. What if you're ready to go faster and you don't realize it? Being tied to the watch can sometimes be a hindrance to progress.

For 20 x 400 meters, you'll quickly learn if you're sustaining a pace that you could mimic for the 5K race. If you're not sure and get to the 20th repeat completely spent, you went too fast. You want to feel like you could do one more if you had to. Only experience can really teach you how to do this.

You can do this workout a couple of times throughout a 10-week training program. It's just one in a plethora of speed sessions to choose from each week. If you're getting antsy for feedback, put the watch on when you do this one for the last time—maybe a week before race day. It'll be a good gauge to see what to expect when you toe the line.

Don't forget to warm up and cool down—I like to jog 15 to 20 minutes before and after the set.

so through some trial and error, you can figure out variations in the suggested schedules that might help you meet your individual goals.

Beginner 5K Training Plan

(Based on 10 weeks of training before the goal race and the assumption that a runner can already comfortably jog 2 miles without walk breaks)

	MONDAY	TUESDAY	WEDNESDAY	
Week 1	2 miles easy	Rest day	2 miles easy	
Week 2	2 miles easy	2 miles easy	Rest day	
Week 3	3 miles easy	2 miles easy + 2 x 20-second strides	Rest day	
Week 4	3 miles easy	3 miles easy + 4 x 20-second strides	Rest day	
Week 5	3 miles easy	3 miles easy + 4 x 20-second strides	Rest day	
Week 6	3 miles easy	4 miles easy	Rest day	
Week 7	4 miles easy	4 miles easy	Rest day	
Week 8	4 miles easy	4 miles easy	Cross-train 30 minutes	
Week 9	3 miles easy	4 miles easy	Rest day	
Week 10	3 miles easy	2 miles easy	Rest day	

Easy = Pace that you can sustain for long periods of time. You could carry on a conversation without any problem at this pace.

Strides = Do these on a flat surface, gradually accelerating to about 90 percent effort. Take full recovery before starting the next one.

THURSDAY	FRIDAY	SATURDAY	SUNDAY
Rest day	Cross-train 30 minutes	3 miles easy	Rest day
Cross-train 30 minutes	Rest day	3 miles easy	Rest day
3 miles easy	Cross-train 30 minutes	4 miles easy	Rest day
Cross-train 30 minutes	2 miles easy	4 miles easy	Rest day
3 miles easy	Cross-train 30 minutes	5 miles easy	Rest day
3 miles easy + 4 x 20-second strides	Cross-train 30 minutes	5 miles easy	Rest day
3 miles easy + 4 x 20-second strides	Cross-train 30 minutes	4 miles easy	Rest day
Rest day	4 miles easy	5 miles easy	Rest day
2 miles easy + 4 x 20-second strides	Cross-train 30 minutes	3 miles easy	Rest day
2 miles easy or cross-train 30 minutes	Rest day	15 minutes easy + 4 x 20-second strides	Race day

Cross-train = Thirty minutes of nonimpact or low-impact aerobic activity, such as cycling, elliptical training, or swimming.

Rest day = Either take off or do 30 minutes of nonimpact or low-impact aerobic activity, such as cycling, elliptical training, or swimming.

Seasoned Runner 5K Training Plan

(Based on 10 weeks of training with experience running up to 40 miles per week)

	MONDAY	TUESDAY	WEDNESDAY	
Week 1	4 miles easy	5 miles easy	Cross-train 60 minutes	
Week 2	5 miles easy	5 miles at slightly faster than easy pace. Find a hilly route.	Cross-train 60 minutes	
Week 3	6 miles easy	5 miles at slightly faster than easy pace	Cross-train 60 minutes	
Week 4	5 miles easy	5 miles: 2 miles easy 10 x 20-second sprints up steep hill (10 percent grade) with jog-down hill recovery between 2 miles easy	Cross-train 60 minutes	
Week 5	6 miles easy	5 miles slightly faster than easy pace. Find a hilly course, if possible, or do the following: 2 miles easy 10 x 20-second sprints up steep hill (10 percent grade) with jog-down hill recovery between 2 miles easy	Cross-train 60 minutes	
Week 6	5 miles easy	7 miles slightly faster than easy pace. Find a hilly route.	Cross-train 60 minutes	

	THURSDAY	FRIDAY	SATURDAY	SUNDAY
	5 miles fartlek: 2-mile warmup 10 x 60 seconds at 5K effort/90 seconds easy 2-mile cooldown	Rest day	4 miles easy	7 miles easy
	5 miles fartlek: 1 mile easy 2 miles of 2 minutes at 5K effort/1 minute easy 2 miles easy	Rest day	4 miles easy	7 miles easy
	6 miles fartlek: 2 miles easy 2 miles of 2 minutes at 5K effort/1 minute easy 2 miles easy	Rest day	4 miles easy	8 miles easy
	7 miles fartlek: 2 miles easy 3 miles of 90 seconds at 5K effort/1 minute easy 2 miles easy	Rest day	5 miles easy	7 miles easy
	7 miles speed workout: 1.5-mile warmup 10 x 400 meters at 5K pace with 200-meter jog between 1.5-mile cooldown	Rest day	6 miles easy	8 miles easy
	8 miles speed workout: 2-mile warmup 6 x 800 meters at 5K pace with 400-meter recovery jog between 2-mile cooldown	Rest day	7 miles easy	9 miles easy

(continued)

Seasoned Runner 5K Training Plan *(cont.)*

	MONDAY	TUESDAY	WEDNESDAY	
Week 7	6 miles easy	8 miles with hills (find a hilly route and run slightly faster than easy pace) OR find a hill with 10 percent grade and do this workout: 2 miles easy 24 x 20-second sprint uphill with jog-down recovery 2 miles easy	Cross-train 60 minutes	
Week 8	6 miles easy	6 miles (find a hilly route or run this slightly faster than easy pace, but not as fast as tempo pace)	Cross-train 60 minutes	
Week 9	4 miles easy	5 miles easy	Cross-train 60 minutes	
Week 10	4 miles easy	4 miles with fartlek: 1 mile easy 2 miles of 1 minute at 5K effort/1 minute easy 1 mile easy	Rest day	

RACING THE 5K

You can approach race day in multiple ways, depending on what your goals are.

FOR BEGINNERS, the objective should be to sustain your pace throughout the 3.1 miles and finish strong. This will require you to not get caught up in the crowds of other runners who will attack that first mile too fast. Remember your easy pace, which will naturally be a little faster on race day because of your adrenaline.

THURSDAY	FRIDAY	SATURDAY	SUNDAY
8 miles speed workout: 2-mile warmup 3 x 1 mile at 5K pace with 800-meter jogs between 2-mile cooldown	Rest day	7 miles easy	9 miles easy
8 miles speed workout: 10–12 x 400 meters at 5K pace with 200-meter recovery jog or walk between 2-mile warmup 2-mile cooldown	Rest day	5 miles easy	8 miles easy
6 miles with fartlek: 1 mile easy 4 miles of 90 seconds at 5K effort/1 minute easy 1 mile easy	Rest day	4 miles easy	8 miles easy
4 miles easy	Rest day	20 minutes easy + 4 x 20-second strides	Race day

Never underestimate the power of pinning on a race number and beginning a run with thousands of anxious athletes just waiting for a gun to go off. Don't panic if that first split is a little quicker than normal, but adjust the pace in the second mile and settle into that rhythm you've practiced over the past 10 weeks. You want to cross the finish line with a positive experience, so you're motivated to keep at it. If you feel like you still have something left in the tank with about three-quarters or half of a mile to go, pick it up

Tackling a 5K Race Series

Many communities offer a series of 5Ks throughout the summer months. Often they're cheap, no-frills events where you can test your fitness or rekindle a rivalry with your running frenemies. The 5K summer series events are always fun, but training for them can be a little tricky. Here are a few tips to peak multiple times in a short window:

1. Look at the schedule of races and pick two that are most important to you. Maybe the series travels to different courses. Which ones cater to your strengths? Plan to shine on those occasions. You can lessen the mileage of your training those weeks and do a bit of a mini-taper to feel a little fresher.

2. Use the other races in the series as your speed workout for those weeks. Don't decrease your mileage during the week to "peak" for these races—just adjust the days of the week so that your speed workout falls on race day.

3. Give yourself enough time. If you're preparing for a season of races, start laying down a solid base beginning 3 months prior. Start with the basics like mileage, then gradually add in the speedwork and sharpening for the 5K as you get closer to the beginning of the series.

4. Don't forget the importance of recovery between races. You want to give yourself every opportunity to rejuvenate, which starts right after each race. Hydrate, refuel, and cool down. If you're feeling fatigued the next day, cut back on planned mileage or consider a day of cross-training. Eat nutritious meals and sleep well—both strategies will keep you healthy and race ready throughout the summer.

a notch and see what you've got, almost like the strides you did each week.

FOR SEASONED RUNNERS, the 5K requires an immediate attention to pace. You can't go out conservatively if you are trying to clock your best time, but you can't go crazy either. It's a fine line at this distance. Start off at a pace that you are certain you can sustain and stay right there for the first mile. In the second mile, you'll start passing all the people who clearly had no race strategy coming in or more likely just didn't follow their plans very well. They'll start falling off their pace, and it'll make you feel like a rock star. Around mile 2.5 you'll notice the people around you—these are your competitors. They're the ones who are going to steal your age group award (that plaque belongs to you!), so it's time to focus on how many of them you can begin to pick off. In the third mile, just keep focusing on runners ahead of you and see how many of them you can catch. If you have any other gears left, it's time to use them. Pour it all out. Finish with nothing left in the tank. Sure, you might throw up. That's acceptable behavior at the finish line; just try to be polite and don't hit your competitors' shoes.

WARMUP AND COOLDOWN. More than longer distances, the 5K requires a decent pre- and postrace routine to get your body primed to perform and then help it begin to recover. Get to the race with at least 60 minutes to spare. For seasoned runners, take that time to get a good jog going for about 20 minutes (if you're a beginner, get a nice 10-minute vigorous walk in). If you usually do dynamic stretching or drills before your workouts, then include those in your routine—I know drills are useful for many runners, though I don't usually do them myself. When there's about 10 minutes until go time, do a few strides—about four of them. After you cross the finish line, grab a drink, walk for a few minutes, then go for another 20-minute jog. You may feel like celebrating instead, but that can wait. You'll allow your muscles to start repairing themselves so that you won't be too sore later. And you'll be ready to train for the next race.

Chapter 4

Training for and Racing 10Ks

Choosing and preparing for a 10K, race strategies, and key workouts

I hold a lot of sentimental attachment to the 10K. It was the first race distance I ever attempted, and it's what got me hooked on this sport. In fact, I'd guess that I've run 300 or more 10Ks in my career. A lot of people seem to neglect the 10K—it sort of gets lost somewhere between the popularity of the 5K and the ambitious goals of the half marathon and marathon. But racing 6.2 miles has a lot of merit for a variety of reasons—there's a lot of running wisdom to be gained in mastering this distance. To be sure, it taught me a lot in my early days of racing.

I always liked to use the 10K as a gauge of fitness while training for longer distances or as a way to infuse a bit of faster running into my routine so that my legs don't lose touch with that quicker turn-over that can deteriorate when focused on longer races. You don't want to become a permanent shuffler. Many runners use it as a tool in prepping for other goals. When Meb Keflezighi won the silver medal at the 2004 Athens Olympic marathon, he won the 10,000 meters at the US Olympic Trials just a few weeks beforehand, as did Deena Kastor on her way to the bronze medal in the women's marathon at the 2004 Games. If it worked for them, then perhaps there's something to it? Racing the faster 6.2 miles leading up to a longer "A" race makes that marathon (or half marathon) goal pace seem much easier. In fact, 10K pace should be 30 to 35 seconds faster than marathon pace.

For those who are a bit newer to running and have a few 5K races under their belts, the next natural step in running progression is the 10K, of course. I can't emphasize enough that I believe beginner runners should take all of these steps before eyeing the marathon, thought I know many just jump to 26.2 miles with no consequences. Trying out the 5K and 10K is a great way to safely and gradually increase volume in training, get used to speed workouts, and learn more about pacing. Plus, if you already have a baseline level of fitness from training for that 5K, it should only take a quick 8 weeks to get ready to tackle a debut 6.2-mile race.

There are so many 10K events worth running. The Bolder Boulder, in Boulder, Colorado, has become a beacon for the start of summer racing each Memorial Day weekend, with 54,000 runners finishing each year. The race is made even more exciting because the elites have a separate start, making it easy to watch them compete. They join together for the international team challenge, adding a fun twist on the competition. The race finishes on Folsom Field inside the University of Colorado's stadium, which fills with about 50,000 screaming fans. Not many finish lines can rival that kind of enthusiasm in the United States, and it's inspirational to see so many people display such enthusiasm for the professionals and the sport in general. The Memorial Day program afterward on the field is also touching and meaningful.

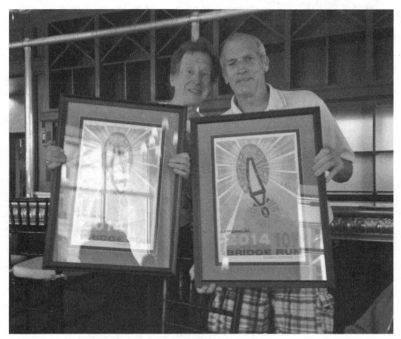

Bill Rodgers (left) and Bart receive commemorative gifts at the 2014 Cooper River Bridge Run.

But one of my favorite 10Ks is the Cooper River Bridge Run in Charleston, South Carolina, which is usually held in the beginning of April. It's the third-largest 6.2-mile race in the country and the fifth-largest road race in the United States, with about 40,000 participants each year. Back when I ran it, the truss bridge was this rickety old structure that I swear swayed back and forth with so many people running over it. I'm pretty sure I felt some movement that wasn't natural. You'd see some runners with visible fear on their faces as they felt the vibrations, wondering if it was safe or if the whole thing was going to crash under the pressure of thousands of runners. In fact, I remember many of the professional athletes at Cooper River staying right in the middle of that bridge because they were, just like almost everybody else, a little scared of it. I always wondered how cars could have ever safely passed over it, but they

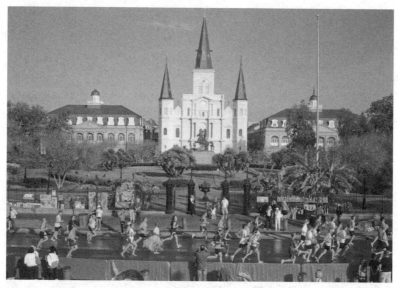

The party never ends in New Orleans. Runners find bunny costumes and adult beverages everywhere.

did, which gave me a little reassurance that we'd all get to the other side without catastrophe. You could see down to the water below through the trusses—it was just part of the charm and mystique of this popular race back then.

Since that time, a beautiful new bridge has been built, which opened in 2005, connecting Charleston and Mount Pleasant. It's a work of art. It's about 2.5 miles long, so you spend a good portion of the race on it, and the views are spectacular. It's a point-to-point course, with a slight uphill as you go over the first half of the bridge and then the inevitable downhill as you make your way to the other side. After you get off the bridge and head into downtown Charleston, it's as flat as flat can be to the finish line. When you are done, be prepared to join the finish festival party, where you'll find plenty of refreshments and people ready to celebrate. Charleston is a great destination and a fun area to visit. As you might imagine, there's a lot of southern hospitality on display, plus it has access to beaches and many historical landmarks worth checking out.

I guess I must gravitate to the South for my choice of 10K races, because over the years I've also enjoyed the Crescent City Classic, which is held in New Orleans and dubbed the CCC 10K. It's also a springtime event, held Easter weekend each year. The CCC is about as flat a course as you'll ever find so, minus a few turns, it's a fast course and the atmosphere is classic New Orleans. Get ready to party. Prepare for a combination of road racing and Mardi Gras partying all rolled into one. While the elite field zips through at breakneck speed, the middle and back of the pack have the option of taking a less serious approach. The party never ends in New Orleans. Runners find bunny costumes and adult beverages everywhere. You'll also find the usual water and sports drinks out there, if that's more your style.

The CCC starts downtown in front of the Superdome, then goes through the French Quarter and up Esplanade Avenue to New Orleans City Park, where—you guessed it—a huge party awaits. That's when the fun really begins. Beer is served along with jambalaya and all kinds of Creole cuisine. I'm a sucker for these kinds of races that truly embrace the regional culture and give runners a sense of it at their events. People really go a little crazy at the end of this 6.2 miles—it's about as close to a Bourbon Street atmosphere as you're going to find at a race. And who can resist andouille sausage after a hard effort? The aroma is delicious—if I weren't a vegetarian, I would devour it.

BART'S TAKE ON THE PEACHTREE ROAD RACE

At least one time in your road-racing career I highly recommend that you kick off the Fourth of July in Atlanta at the Peachtree Road

Race 10K. With 60,000 participants, it's the largest road race in the country and now an Independence Day tradition. The race always attracts a top-notch professional field as well.

Your fate at Peachtree depends on how well you can negotiate all kinds of variables like weather and huge crowds. It's July. It's Atlanta. It's going to be hot and humid. It might even rain. Nobody really can say for sure what to expect until they line up—and the earlier waves may experience completely different conditions than the final waves. If you're agoraphobic, this probably isn't the race for you. If you don't know if you're agoraphobic, you'll find out pretty quickly that day. But this race organization can handle it—the officials have the logistics down pat and the event goes remarkably smoothly, especially when you consider how many people they're trying to move safely over 6.2 miles.

Unless you're a member of the professional field or seeded in one of the first corrals, you'll be slowed at the start by the sheer number of runners around you. Don't panic and start trying to "frogger"

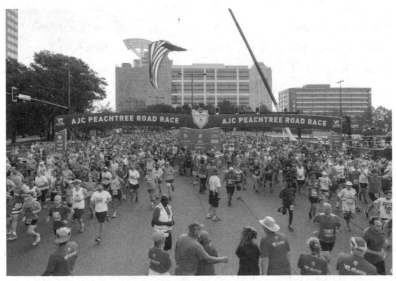

The Peachtree Road Race is an Independence Day tradition, with plenty of people packing the hot streets of Atlanta.

your way around people. All the weaving in and out and across the road is only going to add time and waste energy—it will also add distance. Be patient. Sometimes it's even helpful in the 10K to have a more conservative start to assure a stronger finish. The road will open up within the first mile and you'll find space to get on your pace.

Peachtree has a reputation for being a bit hilly, but it is a net-downhill course, so keep that in mind when you're scaling what's known as Cardiac Hill, which, appropriately enough, is located right in front of Piedmont Hospital. The thing about this ascent is that you've been gently coasting downhill for the first 3 miles of the race by the time you hit it. You're probably hot at this point, and all of a sudden you are facing a 200-foot climb over three-quarters of a mile. Keep the same effort up the hill instead of trying to force the same pace.

Peachtree isn't an event where many will set a personal record, but it is possible to do so if that's your goal. The reason to run this one, however, is to savor the experience. If you read and follow the directions that the race officials provide on the Web site regarding transportation and logistics, you'll have a smooth, enjoyable day, and that will likely be reflected in your results. The energy of the spectators is infectious—very few points on the course aren't lined with fans offering high fives and cheers.

Racing Tips for Peachtree

➤ **TRY TO ACCLIMATE TO RUNNING IN WARM CONDITIONS.**
While not everybody lives in a place that has the temperatures or the humidity level of an Atlanta summer day, you can work with what you've got. If Peachtree is your goal race, plan to run at the warmest part of the day once or twice a week. If you're not able to fit that into your work schedule, then try to do a few of your speed

Handling Heat and Humidity on Race Day

One race-day variable that I see runners struggle with over and over again is the weather. They don't seem to understand that the temperature isn't something they can control, but how they adjust to it is completely their call. If the race is hot, as Peachtree and sometimes the Monument Avenue 10K usually are, you can adapt your expectations and still emerge with a positive experience.

Here are my tips for dealing with a hot and humid race day.

1. **Adjust expectations.**
   Don't start the race with the same goals you had in mind when you were training. If you stubbornly go after the same pace you practiced, you'll probably end up on a death march toward the finish line. Begin conservatively and figure out if you're able to gradually step on the gas over the final few miles. And allow yourself to set different goals if the conditions just aren't cooperating. Studies show that for every 5°F that temperatures rise after 60°, you can expect to slow down nearly 20 to 30 seconds per mile. Forget the watch and run by perceived effort. You'll probably finish

workouts or some of the weekend long runs during times that the temperatures are highest. That way your body won't be in total shock on the Fourth of July.

➤ **PRACTICE HYDRATION.** Train your gut to accept fluids before your run and a couple of times during your run, if needed. If you're racing a 10K in cooler conditions, chances are you won't always need to use aid stations during the race if you've hydrated much stronger that way.

2. **Wear appropriate clothing.** You want to make sure your gear is helping to keep you cool, so pull out loosely fitting apparel made of sweat-wicking material. Consider wearing sunglasses and a cap, and apply sunscreen.

3. **Splash yourself.** When you pass aid stations, take a cup to drink and a cup to splash water over your head as a cooling mechanism. Sometimes races will provide other cooling measures, like cold sponges or hoses spraying the runners. If you feel like you're overheating, take advantage of those amenities.

4. **Hydrate before, during, and after the race.** You want your urine to be light yellow—that's how you know your hydration game is on point. Make sure you're taking in a couple of ounces of sports drinks that contain electrolytes, which help your body absorb water. There's no need to overdo it, but make sure you aren't feeling thirsty. You want to pay attention to your hydration beginning the day before the race.

adequately beforehand. But a race in the summer in the South is a different ball game, especially one where many participants are held up at the start line behind thousands of others, extending your time out in the toasty elements.

➤ **PLAN YOUR PRERACE FUELING.** Just because the start time is advertised as 7:30 a.m. doesn't mean most runners are actually starting at that time. The final wave actually goes off more than

90 minutes later. So look at what time your corral is slated to begin and work backward from there to figure out when to eat breakfast. You'll probably need to pack some fuel to eat when you arrive. You can practice this eating routine during training, preferably when you do your weekend long runs, so you know the timing and what foods agree with your system.

BART'S FAVORITE 10K: MONUMENT AVENUE

The 10K that I most look forward to is Monument Avenue in Richmond, Virginia, which also takes place at the end of March or the beginning of April. As the race organization describes it: "A pep rally. A block party. A race. A gateway to fitness." That about covers it.

The course is basically a giant out-and-back on Monument Avenue, which is a famous stretch of tree-lined road with a beautiful grassy mall dividing it. At this time of year, the blossoms are coming out, which makes the view spectacular. Along the avenue are statues of Confederates of the Civil War, including Robert E. Lee, Jefferson Davis, and "Stonewall" Jackson. Arthur Ashe, the tennis star and humanitarian, is also memorialized here—he was a native of Richmond.

What I really enjoy about this race is that the field of 30,000 people is divided into around 30 or more waves based on pace, starting every 3 minutes, so you're racing people who are of the same ability level. There are waves that require proof of qualification, then there are other groups dedicated to walkers or those who may not have much running experience yet. If you are hoping to race with a group of friends, you can do so just by starting in the wave of the slowest runner. It creates a good atmosphere that accommodates all kinds of goals—from those who are there to clock a personal record to those

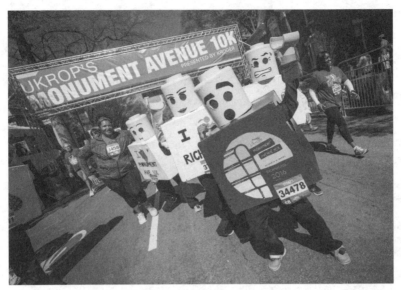

When Bart is helping with television commentary, the costumes at the Monument Avenue 10K often stump him.

who just want to have fun or have set a goal to finish the distance. And 20 live bands are out on the course just for good measure and added motivation, which certainly uplifts the atmosphere (20 bands in just 6.2 miles is a lot of music).

The race also offers prizes for subcompetitions. For example, one runner is selected to have a head start on the pro field (based on ability level). If that person beats the winner, he or she is awarded $2,500. The runners aren't the only competitors, either—the race offers a spirit award to the best group of fans on the course. There's even a "porch party" award for the people who live on the avenue and throw the best spectating fiesta.

The Monument Avenue race might also showcase one of the biggest arrays of costumed runners I've ever seen. Volunteers judge the costumes and award cash prizes for individuals and groups. I think this part of the event has actually presented the most challenging part of my job when I help with the television broadcast commentary. I think I know pop culture well until somebody dressed up as a Pokémon character crosses the finish line and I don't know what that person is supposed to be. Often people dress as pop icons or people who are currently in the news, and I don't always get it, which can be funny when I'm on live television.

All of this together, on a great flat course, makes this a truly unique community event. You can run fast, and you can also absorb the enthusiasm of the crowd.

Racing Tips for Monument Avenue

➤ **YOU'LL RUN ON COBBLESTONES.** Just beware that for a portion of the race you'll run on cobblestones, which is not a big deal because they are pretty smooth. You can't prepare for this, unless you also happen to live in an area that has cobblestone streets, but it helps to know you'll encounter an uneven surface around mile five. A lot of people hardly notice the difference, but some do.

➤ **THE WEATHER IS UNPREDICTABLE.** Sometimes it's unseasonably warm and humid. Other times it's rainy and chilly. Spring in Virginia is a mixed bag. Prepare to be surprised and adjust for whatever Mother Nature throws at you.

➤ **YOU MAY EXPERIENCE A HEADWIND.** It's possible on a breezy day that on a big out-and-back course you'll feel the wind hit your face in one half or the other. Check which way the wind is blowing before you start so you won't be surprised (or disappointed) at the turnaround if you feel a little added resistance on the way home.

➤ **THE FIRST HALF IS SLIGHTLY UPHILL.** The grade is so minimal and hard to notice visually, you may not even realize that you're going slightly uphill during the first part of the race. Also, you'll be feeling fresh coming off that starting line, which will probably minimize the effect. Hopefully you'll notice that you're going downhill on the way to the finish, though.

➤ **PLAN TO RUN EVEN SPLITS.** This is a great course to get into a groove early and stay there. When you turn around at 3 miles, just keep pressing at your goal pace. As with any race, don't get caught up with the adrenaline-powered fast starters—remember that you'll catch them when they start fading. Get on your goal pace early and stay there, clicking off 1 mile at a time.

HOW TO TRAIN FOR 10KS

The 10K requires a little bit of everything—6.2 miles is long enough to demand endurance and strength, but short enough to also command speed. No wonder most people skip right over it in favor of a more defined distance. This one can be tricky—there's no doubt about it.

To prepare for the 10K, the typical ingredients are needed after a solid base of fitness is built: the long run of up to 10 miles for more seasoned runners and around 7 or 8 for newer people; the speed workouts in the form of hills, tempo runs, and track workouts; and a slightly higher volume of easy runs each week than is required for the 5K. If you're going for a 10K personal best, you have to implement some pace-specific work into your weekly routine, too.

The training plans that follow are suggestions—as I said before, all runners are different, and no one training plan fits all needs. Always listen to your body and make adjustments based on how you're responding to your schedule.

Beginner 10K Training Plan

(Before beginning this 8-week schedule, the runner should be able to comfortably complete a 5K.)

	MONDAY	TUESDAY	WEDNESDAY	
Week 1	3 miles easy	Rest day	2 miles easy	
Week 2	Rest day	3 miles easy	3 miles easy	
Week 3	3 miles easy	2 miles easy + 2 x 20-second strides	Rest day	
Week 4	Rest day	3 miles easy + 4 x 20-second strides	3 miles easy	
Week 5	3 miles easy	Rest day	3 miles easy + 4 x 20-second strides	
Week 6	Rest day	3 miles easy	Rest day	
Week 7	4 miles easy	3 miles easy	Rest day	
Week 8	3 miles easy	3 miles easy	Cross-train 30 minutes	

Easy = Pace that you can sustain for long periods of time. You could carry on a conversation without any problem at this pace.

Strides = Do these on a flat surface, gradually accelerating to about 90 percent effort. Take full recovery before starting the next one.

THURSDAY	FRIDAY	SATURDAY	SUNDAY
Rest day	Cross-train 30 minutes	3 miles easy	3 miles easy
Cross-train 30 minutes	3 miles easy	Rest day	4 miles easy
3 miles easy	Cross-train 30 minutes	4 miles easy	5 miles easy
Cross-train 30 minutes	4 miles easy	Rest day	6 miles easy
3 miles easy	Cross-train 30 minutes	3 miles easy	7 miles easy
4 miles easy + 4 x 20-second strides	3 miles easy	Cross-train 30 minutes	6 miles easy
3 miles easy + 4 x 20-second strides	Rest day	Cross-train 30 minutes	4 miles easy
3 miles easy	Rest day	15 minutes easy + 4 x 20-second strides	Race day

Cross-train = Thirty minutes of nonimpact or low-impact aerobic activity, such as cycling, elliptical training, or swimming.

Seasoned Runner 10K Training Plan

(Assumes runner has a base of 20 miles per week and at least 5K racing experience)

	MONDAY	TUESDAY	WEDNESDAY	
Week 1	5 miles easy	5 miles easy	Cross-train 60 minutes	
Week 2	5 miles easy	6 miles at slightly faster than easy pace	Cross-train 60 minutes	
Week 3	6 miles easy	6 miles at slightly faster than easy pace	Cross-train 60 minutes	
Week 4	6 miles easy	5 miles: 2 miles easy 10 x 20-second sprints up steep hill (10 percent grade) with jog-down recovery between 2 miles easy	Cross-train 60 minutes	

THURSDAY	FRIDAY	SATURDAY	SUNDAY
6 miles fartlek: 2-mile warmup 12 x 60 seconds at 5K effort/ 90 seconds easy 2-mile warmdown	Rest day	4 miles easy	7 miles easy
6 miles with hill intervals: 2 miles easy 6 x 1-minute uphill sprints (pick a hill that is gradual, not steep) with jog-down recovery 2 miles easy	Rest day	4 miles easy	8 miles easy
7 miles speed workout: 2-mile warmup 6 x 400 meters at slightly slower than 5K pace with 200-meter float between 2-mile cooldown	Rest day	4 miles easy	9 miles easy
8 miles speed workout: 2-mile warmup 4 x 1 mile at 10K pace with 1 minute rest between 2-mile cooldown	Rest day	5 miles easy	9 miles easy

(continued)

Seasoned Runner 10K Training Plan *(cont.)*

	MONDAY	TUESDAY	WEDNESDAY	
Week 5	6 miles easy	5 miles slightly faster than easy pace. Find a hilly course.	Cross-train 60 minutes	
Week 6	5 miles easy	6 miles with hill intervals: 2 miles easy 6 x 1-minute uphill sprints (pick a hill that is gradual, not steep) with jog-down recovery 2 miles easy	Cross-train 60 minutes	
Week 7	5 miles easy	5 miles easy	Cross-train 60 minutes	
Week 8	5 miles easy	4 miles with fartlek: 1 mile easy 2 miles of 1 minute at 5K effort/1 minute easy 1 mile easy	Rest day	

THURSDAY	FRIDAY	SATURDAY	SUNDAY
7 miles speed workout: 2.5-mile warmup 6 x 400 meters at slightly slower than 5K pace with 200-meter float between 2.5-mile cooldown	Rest day	6 miles easy	8 miles easy
8 miles speed workout: 2-mile warmup 6 x 800 meters at 5K pace with 400-meter recovery jog between 2-mile cooldown	Rest day	7 miles easy	10 miles easy
6 miles speed workout: 2 miles easy 3 x 1 mile at 10K pace with 2 minutes recovery 1 mile easy	Rest day	4 miles easy	6 miles easy
4 miles easy	Rest day	20 minutes easy + 4 x 20-second strides	Race day

Bart's Key 10K Workouts

I'm a firm believer that every 10K workout for experienced runners should include 3 miles of quality work, meaning that when you add up the time you spent at a prescribed pace, you should be near 3 miles.

Although you don't necessarily have to use the track to achieve great workouts, visiting the big oval is my preference for the 10K distance.

Workout:

20-minute warmup jog

6–8 x 400 meters at 5K pace with 200-meter "float" between each interval (the 200 meters is not a walk or a jog—it's a little bit faster than that)

15-minute cooldown jog

Why: This workout was made famous by Australian marathoner Rob de Castella, and there are many variations of it you can construct for yourself (try 3 sets of 1200 meters/400 meters at 10K pace with 100 meters float between, for example). You won't fully recover during that 200 meters, so the pace will feel challenging as the workout goes on—it's important to make sure you don't start out the first intervals too fast. This is almost like a fartlek run, but a little more structured. Besides teaching you proper pacing, it also trains your muscles to more effectively use lactate.

When: This workout should be placed into your portfolio of weekly speed sessions only after you've built a proper base of mileage and your fitness level is good. You can schedule it every other week, but you should not do it the week leading up to your goal race.

Workout:

20-minute warmup jog

4 x 1 mile at 10K pace with 1 minute rest in between

20-minute cooldown jog

Why: This one is just simple and classic, but you can get a lot of benefits out of it for the 10K. First of all, you learn what the effort of your goal pace feels like. Again, the short rest is key to reaping the benefits of the workout, though that minute might mentally make the work more manageable than simply running 4 miles at 10K pace. Remember to keep the pace at your current 10K ability level and resist the temptation to go faster. **When:** This is the kind of workout you can do once a week without risk of injury. You should either shorten the length of the intervals or the duration of the workout during the week of your race. You can also go up to 6 x 1 mile after you've mastered the 4 x 1 mile to ramp up your intensity during your training cycle.

Workout:

20-minute warmup jog

8 x 1-minute sprints uphill (not too steep) with jog back down as recovery

20-minute cooldown jog

Why: Hills are great for building strength: They reinforce proper form and they rarely introduce injuries. They're a wonderful way for newer runners to incorporate weekly speedwork.
When: Hills can be done once a week, anytime. Cut down the number of repeats or do not schedule this workout the week leading up to your race.

HOW TO RACE A 10K

When you step up to the 10K from the 5K, it becomes important to break down the distance into manageable chunks that are easier for your mind to chew on. Some like to think about one 5K at a time. Others like to think about 2 miles at a time and set goals for each of those phases of the race. Whatever you do, try to pick a strategy that makes the distance of the race less overwhelming to you.

What I learned in my first few 10K races back in the day is that the race is long enough that you cannot recover if you go out too fast. I clearly remember that first time my brother George lured me to the starting line. I bolted out with the leaders when the gun went off, and I thought I was going to vomit before I hit the halfway point. George, with much more experience, sailed right past me because he obviously knew the perils of bad pacing. It was such a rookie mistake, though one that taught me a lot about the distance—everybody has a few just like that. Those are the most valuable experiences for figuring out how to race. I try to focus on clocking the first mile about 5 or 10 seconds slower than my goal pace. If you think in those terms, you're likely to hit your desired pace because although you're perceiving that you're holding yourself back, you probably aren't actually going that slow—few people are honestly able to be that conservative at the beginning of a race.

The first 2 miles should feel good—not too difficult. If you're already feeling strained, you should back off because the middle miles are the ones you need to nail in order to get that shiny new personal record. It's in miles three, four, and five that the race will get tricky—those are the make-or-break moments. Although you have more leeway in correcting bad pacing than you do in the 5K, it's still pretty critical that you don't let yourself wander too far off your goal. You hit that halfway milestone and get a jolt of energy or at least mentally key off the fact that you're on your way home now. It's time to notice who's around you and if they're slowing down. Check yourself and make sure you're not getting lulled into their declining performance. Typically, many people will start experiencing fatigue at this point, so if you've played your cards right, you should start passing people. Start looking for people ahead of you to pass.

During the last 1.2 miles, it's time to channel all the workouts you completed. Remember how awful you felt toward the end of most of them, but somehow you still finished them? That's what you have to call on here to sustain your cadence. Again, try to reel in runners slightly ahead of you. Once you pass somebody, pick another target to go after. If you have a final gear—and, hopefully, you do—use it in the final half mile of the race.

Just like the 5K, it's important to warm up for the race and prime the body for the quick pace from the gun. If you start a race like the 10K cold, you will have a hard time getting to your pace quick enough. I suggest a 20-minute jog for experienced runners, followed by any dynamic stretching that you do in training, and then 4 x 20-second strides as close to the start time as you can manage. After the race is over, go for another 15-minute cooldown jog—your body will thank you tomorrow. Refuel, hydrate, and get a good night's rest. All of this is critical to repairing your muscles and getting back to the grind. If you've used the race as a tune-up for a longer-distance goal, such as a half marathon or marathon, you'll want to do everything you can to get back to training as soon as you can.

If you're a newer runner, you should still warm up a bit before the race. Go for a brisk 10-minute walk and do three or four 20-second strides before you hit your corral. If you're able, try to do another 10-minute walk when you're finished, but most importantly, start rehydrating and get some rest.

Chapter 5

Training for and Racing Half Marathons

Choosing and preparing for a half marathon, race strategies, and key workouts

The 13.1-mile race is my distance of choice these days. As John Bingham, a former columnist at *Runner's World,* once said: It's twice the fun in half the distance (of the marathon). I find many reasons to love the half marathon, including the fact that there seem to be so many of them to choose from—according to Running USA statistics, there are about 2,700 half marathons offered in the United States and a little less than 2 million finishers each year.

I did my first half marathon in 1980, and back then it wasn't even called a half marathon—it was called a "mini," and there weren't that many of them in existence. A few years later, however, I discovered the Philadelphia Distance Run in its infancy, which is now the Rock 'n' Roll Philadelphia Half Marathon. It became one of my most beloved events each year, only about 60 minutes from where I live. But it goes to show that the running industry for a long time wasn't even sure what to name the half marathon.

Perhaps it wasn't as widely regarded because it isn't contested in the Olympics (though there is continually chatter about adding it one of these years), unlike most other mainstream distances such as the 5K, 10K, and marathon. To me, although I don't consider it just a half of something else, its name still fits. I've heard that people want to change it to all sorts of different monikers because it insinuates that completing the distance is somehow a lesser achievement, but I say leave it alone. It *is* half of a marathon, but it also is a whole distance worthy of training for. Finishing one is always an accomplishment, and not half of an accomplishment, either.

Runners need to conquer the half marathon before moving on to racing marathons—but I often see successful first-timers then immediately move to 26.2 miles. And in order to get faster at the marathon, it behooves experienced runners to first get faster at the half. The distance is a good predictor of how you might do at 26.2 miles. And for those who are juggling busy careers, families, and other commitments, the half takes far less time in preparation, but plenty of training that it is still quite an achievement. It's the best of both worlds, but the half marathon is not all-consuming and presents less risk for injury, too.

Many marathon events have gained in popularity and participation by adding the 13.1-mile option—which often sells out faster than the original 26.2-mile distance. I applaud the events that come up with a twist, such as the San Francisco Marathon in July, where runners can choose the first half (scenic, across the Golden Gate Bridge) or the second half (flatter, with better chance of a best time).

I'll always remember the Miami Half Marathon in January, which I've run a couple of times. It starts around 6:15 a.m., when it is still dark outside. When I ran, by the time we headed over to South Beach, you'd see all these people coming out of nightclubs who hadn't even gone home to bed yet. They would try to get into their cars at 7 a.m. and the streets would be closed down, the roads flooded with thousands of runners. It was awesome—it was this confluence of healthy people who went to bed at 9 p.m. and partiers who never went to sleep. Quite different lifestyles, but the scene was priceless. The "clubbers" were stuck, so they cheered us on.

But not all 13.1-mile races are a hit because they are attached to the longer race. The Brooklyn Half Marathon, from New York Road Runners, is the largest in the country, with about 27,000 entrants, and in 2017 it sold out in 26 minutes. It's probably easier to get Beyoncé concert tickets. Why do so many people want to experience Brooklyn? You run through Prospect Park, through the heart of the historic borough, past the Brooklyn Museum, along Ocean Parkway, and get to finish on the famous Coney Island boardwalk, which I think is the biggest attraction of all. Beach, boardwalk, hot dogs, beers, roller coasters—after running a half marathon, what more could you want? While the first part of the course has a couple of minor hills, the last half is flat and fast.

Whether you're going for an experience or for a fast time, you can certainly find your perfect race easily. The key is to look at the calendar and make sure you have adequate time to prepare, especially if it's your first 13.1-mile race. If you have a baseline of running fitness already, it will take about 10 weeks to be ready to cover the distance. If you're using it as a tune-up for a marathon, it's best to schedule it about 3 or 4 weeks out from your main event.

(continued on page 71)

Tips for First-Time Half Marathoners

If it's your first stab at 13.1 miles, it's going to be a great step in your running journey. However, moving up to this distance also presents a few more things to think about in your training and during the race. Learning how to hydrate, fuel, and recover are more important than ever—and it's smart to learn how to do all of this now, before you consider running a marathon, if that happens to be your ultimate goal.

A few key points to consider:

1. **It's all about the base.** If you've already been consistently training and tried a few 5K and 10K races, you've probably also built up a base of running fitness. Before embarking on the half-marathon plan, make sure you've already built up to running at least three times a week and can comfortably cover about 15 miles in a 7-day period. If you're not there yet, that's okay. Gradually and safely build to it and sustain it for about 3 weeks before you start adding in mileage and speed workouts. Consistency is the key to long-term success, so take all the time you need to safely get to a spot that you can take on more. You shouldn't be in a rush to get there. Long-distance running requires patience.

2. **Long runs are longer.** While you won't need to build the entire way up to 13.1 miles in training, you will learn how to cover up to 11 or 12 miles at one time. If you follow a well-constructed plan, that will occur gradually and at an easy pace—you should be able to carry on a conversation at this speed. Many new runners wonder why they shouldn't cover the entire race distance at least once before the big day. The reason is because 13 miles is likely too much time on your feet at this point. And you don't need to run that far in order to have confidence on race day that you have the ability to finish. If you can run 11 miles, you'll be able to run a half marathon. Trust me.

3. **Find some fuel.** Now that your

long runs are getting longer, it will be time to experiment with your prerun fueling. You'll have to practice what to eat for breakfast before your long runs, and at what time. I don't recommend skipping breakfast. While it may feel uncomfortable at first, you are going to need the calories to get through your run, so training your system to accept that is part of your training. Nutrition and fueling is highly individualized, so start experimenting early to figure out what works for you. Typically a breakfast of easily digestible carbohydrates with a little bit of protein (250 to 300 calories), plus water, about 2 hours before you begin running should do it. But again, this is one part of running you have to figure out for yourself because often what works for your friends will not work for you.

4. **Hydrate along the way.** As your runs become longer, you will likely have to take in water and/or sports drinks while you run. There are plenty of hydra-tion devices on the market—from handheld bottles to vests with bladders in them. Some runners live in areas with water fountains readily available or can stash bottles along the way in the bushes. Remember that hydration will play a significant role in sustaining you and keeping you healthy, too.

5. **You might need snacks.** The longer the run or race, the more necessary it will be to replenish your glycogen stores along the way so you don't run into the dreaded "wall," otherwise known as "bonking." If you're going to be running for 60 minutes or more, consider taking in 30 to 60 grams of carbs while you're out there, spread out every 20 minutes, for example. The market is full of every kind of endurance sports fuel you can think of. The trick is to figure out how much *you* need and what agrees with *your* stomach. Gels are the most convenient and usually contain electrolytes as well. I'd caution against consuming sports drinks *and* gels at the same

(continued)

Tips for First-Time Half Marathoners (cont.)

time—it's more carbohydrate than your body needs at one time and often leads to GI distress because the combination is high in simple sugars. If you're taking in gels or chews, wash them down with plain water instead to avoid a bad gut experience.

6. **Eat after your hard runs.** Within 30 minutes of a hard effort that lasts an hour or more, it's important to eat something to begin the recovery and repair process. Try to consume something that has a 3:1 carb/protein ratio and is about 250 calories. This is to help your body start to replenish itself and repair muscle tissue. It's only a snack—your next meal should be something healthy and nutritious with a nice mix of carbohydrates and protein to continue the process.

7. **Get more sleep.** The more you're running each week, the more important it is to get proper rest. When you're sleeping, your body is given the chance to repair itself and adapt to the increased workload you're putting on it. Don't skimp on the sleep. If you're overtired, you're more likely to get sick or injured, taking you out of training completely. Again, the most critical factor in advancing your running is consistency. You can't build that consistency if you're ill or hurt.

8. **Have a dress rehearsal.** After you've spent 10 weeks figuring out the timing, fuel, and hydration, while teaching your body to cover the miles, make sure your last long run is a dress rehearsal for race day. Get up at the time you plan to wake for the race, eat the same breakfast, head out for the run wearing what you plan to wear on race day (especially the shoes), and practice the fueling and hydration plan you will use. If something goes wrong or doesn't feel right, don't panic. That's the point of the rehearsal—you can fix any kinks before your big day. You're also running long enough now that you may have found some hot spots on your body that chafe. Lube those areas up with Vaseline or other products on the market designed to prevent those painful experiences.

BART'S FAVORITE HALF MARATHON: THE PHILADELPHIA DISTANCE RUN (NOW THE ROCK 'N' ROLL PHILADELPHIA HALF MARATHON)

I have a soft spot for the Philly Distance Run (PDR), which became a Rock 'n' Roll event in 2010. Long before it was bought by the Competitor Group, it was the beloved PDR, and it was one of the first half marathons I ever ran.

In the late 1970s, the PDR attracted some iconic running talent. It was where Lasse Virén ran and won. He was a legend at the time—a distance runner from Finland who had four Olympic gold medals to his name. Joan Benoit Samuelson, the 1984 Olympic marathon gold medalist (the first time women raced the distance at the Games), won it three consecutive times from 1983 to 1985, setting the world record in the half marathon twice. In later iterations of the race, Deena Kastor set the American record on the course. Kim Smith, from New Zealand, ran the fastest women's half marathon on American soil here in a blazing 1:07:11.

To put it plainly, this half marathon, which usually takes place in mid-September (unless somebody like the Pope is visiting, which he did in 2015, so the race was rescheduled for October), has the makings of a fast race for everybody. And for those who are training for a fall marathon, it's perfectly placed on the calendar for a tune-up race. If you're planning to run the Philadelphia Marathon in November, all the more reason to check this one out.

What I enjoy about this course is not only that it's flat and speedy, though those are attractive attributes in any race. It starts on the Benjamin Franklin Parkway, then through a bit of Center City Philly. You run past a lot of history along the way—City Hall, the Museum of Art, and the boathouses on Kelly Drive. It is such a beautiful scene for all these runners to be tucked between the

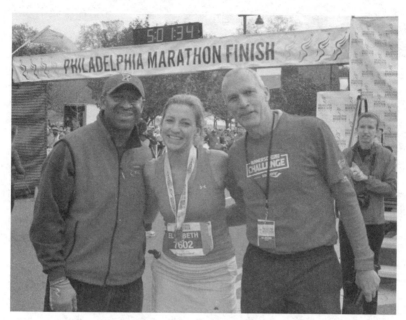

One of Bart's proudest finish-line moments was seeing his niece after running the Philadelphia half marathon.

museum and City Hall—it's so picturesque, in both directions. Philadelphia is where America's first residential street was named. Elfreth's Alley, which is between Second Street and the Delaware River, was where the country's first street addresses originated, dating back to 1702. The Liberty Bell, Betsy Ross's house—all of these amazing pieces of US history are right there in Philadelphia.

When you emerge from downtown, you head to the iconic 8-mile stretch of the course along the river, which utilizes Kelly Drive on the east and Martin Luther King Jr. Drive on the west. It's just classic and the piece that everybody talks about and remembers. There's a bit of an uphill at the end to the finish line, but you only notice it because you've been running on such a flat surface for so long. Your muscles might even welcome the small ascent. You're almost done, so enjoy it.

Race-Day Advice

➤ As with any major city race, parking can be a hassle. If you're not staying in a nearby hotel, plan your parking strategy before race morning and leave yourself plenty of time. The race Web site has an entire transportation and parking section. Read it carefully.

➤ The half marathon has about 16,000 runners and an assigned corral system. Although it takes quite a while for everybody to clear the starting line, don't waste your time weaving around people when you finally hit the road. The streets are wide enough to claim your space. You have 13 miles to settle in, so be patient.

➤ Because it starts at Eakins Oval, space is plentiful to get in a little bit of a warmup before you report to your corral. Make sure you have some time to hit the bathroom line, drop your bag off, and jog for 10 to 15 minutes. Do a few strides to prime your legs for what's to come. Then head to your assigned corral.

➤ This is a great place to shoot for even splits. If you can get on your goal race pace early, and you've trained for it, there is so little variation in terrain that you don't have to make a fancy racing plan to account for hills. The turns are mostly gentle, not hairpins, so they shouldn't be a big factor either.

➤ Save a little something for after the race. You'll definitely want to do your best "Rocky" impersonation, charge up the Art Museum steps, and throw your arms up in victory, just like the movie.

BART'S BABY: THE *RUNNER'S WORLD* HALF MARATHON AND FESTIVAL

When I was asked to help create the *Runner's World* Half Marathon, I wanted to make sure that our event really showcased

Bethlehem, Pennsylvania. Although I've traveled the world, Bethlehem has always been my home. Inviting the running community to where I live is something special, and we designed the 3-day event to celebrate all that is good about our sport—a race for runners, created by runners.

We chose the half-marathon distance because we wanted to present a festival-like atmosphere. If people are arriving to run a marathon, they tend to hibernate and rest in the days beforehand. Then they're too tired to do anything afterward. It's kind of a wash. So we thought the 13.1-mile distance presented a fitting challenge that still allowed visitors to attend the movies, seminars, and workshops we offer without worrying about overdoing it before the race. We also have a 3.8-mile trail run on Friday, a 5K and 10K on Saturday, and then the half marathon on Sunday. Runners can opt for the Hat Trick (5K, 10K, and half), the Five & Dime (5K and 10K), or the Grand Slam (all the races, which conveniently add up to a total of 26.2 miles). There's something for everybody—including kids and

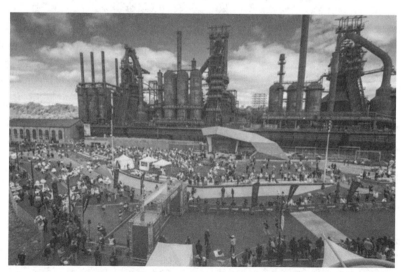

The stacks of Bethlehem Steel are the backdrop of the Runner's World *Half Marathon weekend.*

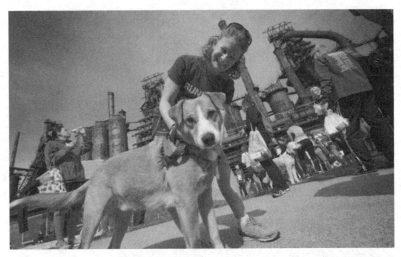

The Runner's World *festival includes a dog race. Here's Marley (with coauthor Erin) after his debut 1 miler.*

dog races. If you're in need of some warm fuzzies and smiles, don't miss the kids and dogs—cuteness abounds.

In 2012 I designed the half-marathon course. Bethlehem is many things—beautiful, scenic, and historic. What it is *not*? Flat. No matter which direction you go, you're going to hit hills. I'd classify our half marathon as "challenging." I like to tell runners that it's pancake flat, but I like blueberries in my pancakes. Some have questioned whether it's more likely I put watermelons in my pancakes. While none of the hills on the course are terribly long or extremely steep, the manner in which they add up can be difficult. But runners don't tend to shy away from a good challenge, so we see a lot of people come back year after year, seeking to do better each time.

But let's talk about other aspects of this race because it certainly offers more than just a lot of hills. It's teeming with US history. You start and finish in the shadow of the former Bethlehem Steel complex. That's where they made the steel that built America. The backbone of our nation was forged right there. You run past original town settlements that date back to 1741, when the Moravians settled on the banks

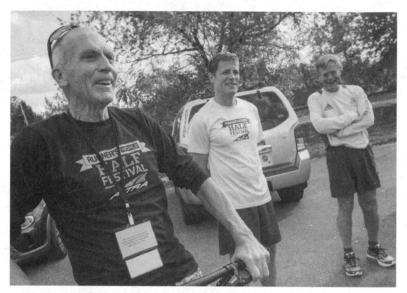

Bart and David Willey, former editor in chief at Runner's World, *enjoy showing off their Bethlehem training ground.*

of Lehigh River and Monocacy Creek. You also pass by Moravian College, founded in 1742 by a 16-year-old girl, Countess Benigna von Zinzendorf. The headquarters for the weekend is the refurbished Bethlehem Steel Mill and ArtsQuest SteelStacks campus.

What also makes this race unique is that all the editors and staff of *Runner's World* are there running, too. They're around all weekend, talking at seminars, signing books, attending the prerace pasta dinner. It's a nice chance to meet the people behind the scenes, who are just as eager to show the world where they run and train. Many of them participate in all the races, too. They're all an integral part of the event and they want to meet their audience, so seek them out and strike up some conversations.

Racing Tips for the *Runner's World* Half Marathon

➤ **PRACTICE HILLS.** More than for most races, I'd recommend implementing a hill workout nearly every week in your training or, better yet, make sure that your long run routes include some nice ascents. And don't forget that practicing running downhill is just as important. After all, what goes up must come down. You'll want to callous those quads for race day (more on downhill running technique and workouts are in Chapter 6).

➤ **START OUT SLOW.** This is a great course to run a negative split (running the second half faster than the first). If you take the first half of the race a few seconds per mile slower than your goal pace, you are setting yourself up to crush the second half, which offers a bit more down than up.

➤ **REMEMBER THESE THREE.** While you'll run into multiple inclines along the way, the course has three main hills to remember. At mile three, the 11th Avenue hill is about one block long. At mile five, it's Schoenersville Road for another half mile uphill. Then at mile seven you'll go up about a quarter mile on Illick's Mill Road.

➤ **EFFORT OVER PACE.** Remember that when facing a rolling course like this, you should focus more on your perceived effort than on the pace you see on your watch. If you maintain that effort on the hills, the pace will take care of itself.

➤ **CARVE OUT SOME TIME ON FRIDAY AND SATURDAY.** Even if you don't intend to run any of the other race distances, you'll want to reserve time to spectate the kids' runs and the dog mile. Trust me. The cuteness factor is out of this world, if I haven't mentioned that already. Children and canines have a special way of reminding us that running is joyful.

➤ **GRAB DINNER WITH THE EDITORS.** How often do you get to enjoy prerace carbs with the editors of *Runner's World*? Probably next to never. Our pasta dinner the night before the race isn't the usual affair. The editors are always on hand, dining among the participants, answering questions, sharing prerace jitters like all runners ready to tackle 13.1 miles.

TRAINING FOR A HALF MARATHON

Preparing for a half marathon is a commitment, but not one that is overwhelming like some of the longer distances can be. For newer runners, increasing mileage gradually will lead to torching more calories and getting even fitter. For experienced runners, the half marathon–specific training can lead to better performance at the longer distances, too, because less mileage will allow for more sharpening and a little more speedwork.

Runners looking to improve speed over the distance should focus more on quality tempo runs during training. These kinds of sessions, when you hold your half-marathon pace for about 3 to 7 miles, will help improve your endurance as well as your capacity to sustain your speed while feeling uncomfortable.

If you're in the camp that will increase mileage by setting a goal to race 13.1 miles, there are a few more things to think about. First, emphasize rest and recovery. You need to allow your body to adapt to the new workload and absorb the work you're putting in. It can only do that properly when you get adequate rest and go down in the mileage for a week every few weeks or so.

Half marathoners also need to pay more heed to nutrition, fueling, and hydration. With more mileage, glycogen stores have to be topped off in order to sustain the workload. Nutritious, whole foods are the best options for your meals. Eating a snack high in carbohydrate with a bit of protein within 30 minutes after a hard effort that lasts 60 minutes or more is critical. And hydration is also important before, during, and after your longer runs. There's no need to overdo the water consumption, but drink enough that you don't feel thirsty and your urine is pale yellow.

For beginner half marathoners, make sure you've built your weekly mileage up to about 15 miles per week before starting a

Bart's Favorite Hill Workout

Training on hills is something I try to do no matter what I'm preparing for. It's a great way to build strength and correct form, and it's a lower-impact form of a speed workout. To get the most out of a hill workout, however, know what the purpose of your session is and don't run something too steep or too fast.

There are a lot of different hill workouts to choose from:

➤ long hill repeats

➤ short hill repeats

➤ hill bounding

➤ downhill strides

Here's a standard one I like to use during half-marathon training, aside from just running on hills during my regular training.

Remember to always warm up and cool down—I prefer about 2 miles each, but if you're looking to add mileage, you can add it there.

1. Find a hill that takes about 2 minutes to run up at a hard pace, not a sprint (it shouldn't be terribly steep, but challenging).

2. Mark off halfway, to indicate a short repeat.

3. Do four sets of short hills, sprinting up to halfway then jogging back down to the bottom.

4. Do four sets of long hills, running hard to the top, jogging to halfway, then sprinting to the bottom. Watch your form in your sprint down by keeping your eyes looking ahead, not down, and leaning slightly forward from your ankles like a ski jumper. When you run down the hill, you don't want to break or lean backward, which can be a natural tendency. Quicken your cadence as you shorten your stride.

5. Do four more sets of short hills.

10-week training plan. Experienced runners should have a base of about 25 miles per week, at least. The rule of thumb is to never increase weekly mileage more than 10 percent each week.

Beginner Half-Marathon Training Plan

(Goal is to complete the 13.1-mile distance [no time goal].)

	MONDAY	TUESDAY	WEDNESDAY	
Week 1	3 miles easy	Rest day	3 miles easy	
Week 2	3 miles easy	Rest day	3 miles easy	
Week 3	Rest day	3 miles easy	4 miles easy + 2 x 20-second strides	
Week 4	Rest day	4 miles easy	3 miles easy + 4 x 20-second strides	
Week 5	3 miles easy	3 miles easy	Rest day	
Week 6	3 miles easy	4 miles easy	Rest day	
Week 7	Rest day	4 miles easy	4 miles easy	
Week 8	Rest day	4 miles easy	5 miles easy + 4 x 20-second strides	
Week 9	3 miles easy	4 miles easy	Rest day	
Week 10	Rest day	4 miles easy	3 miles easy	

Easy = Pace that you can sustain for long periods of time. You could carry on a conversation without any problem at this pace.

Strides = Do these on a flat surface, gradually accelerating to about 90 percent effort. Take full recovery before starting the next one.

Rest day = Either take off or do 30 minutes of nonimpact or low-impact aerobic activity, such as cycling, elliptical training, or swimming.

THURSDAY	FRIDAY	SATURDAY	SUNDAY
Rest day	5 miles easy	Rest day	4 miles easy
4 miles easy	Rest day	3 miles easy	6 miles easy
3 miles easy	Rest day	3 miles easy	7 miles easy
5 miles easy	Rest day	4 miles easy	8 miles easy
5 miles easy	Rest day	5 miles easy	7 miles easy
3 miles easy + 4 x 20-second strides	Cross-train 30 minutes	5 miles easy	10 miles easy
5 miles easy + 4 x 20-second strides	Rest day	4 miles easy	11 miles easy
Rest day	4 miles easy	4 miles easy	10 miles easy
2 miles easy + 4 x 20-second strides	Cross-train 30 minutes	3 miles easy	6 miles easy
3 miles easy	Rest day	20 minutes easy + 4 x 20-second strides	Race day

Seasoned Runner Half-Marathon Training Plan

(Assumes a mileage base of 25 miles per week and previous racing experience of 10K or more)

	MONDAY	TUESDAY	WEDNESDAY	
Week 1	4 miles easy	4 miles easy	Rest day	
Week 2	4 miles easy	4 miles at slightly faster than easy pace. Pick a hilly route.	Rest day	
Week 3	6 miles easy	Rest day	5 miles on hilly terrain	
Week 4	5 miles easy	6 miles: 2 miles easy 12 x 20-second sprints up steep hill (10 percent grade) with jog-down recovery between 2 miles easy	Rest day	
Week 5	6 miles easy	5 miles of hills described in "Bart's Favorite Hill Workout," page 79	Rest day	

THURSDAY	FRIDAY	SATURDAY	SUNDAY
6 miles fartlek: 2-mile warmup 10 x 2 minutes at 10K effort/90 seconds easy 1-mile warmdown	Rest day	4 miles easy	8 miles easy
5 miles fartlek: 1 mile easy 2 miles of 2 minutes at 5K effort/1 minute easy 2 miles easy	Rest day	5 miles easy	9 miles easy
8 miles pace workout: 2 miles easy 3 miles at half-marathon pace 3 miles easy	Rest day	6 miles easy	10 miles easy
8 miles pace workout: 2 miles easy 4 miles at half-marathon pace 2 miles easy	Rest day	6 miles easy	12 miles easy
9 miles speed workout: 2 miles easy 5 miles at half-marathon pace 2 miles easy	Rest day	6 miles easy	13 miles easy

(continued)

Seasoned Runner Half-Marathon Training Plan *(cont.)*

	MONDAY	TUESDAY	WEDNESDAY
Week 6	5 miles easy	Rest day	6 miles with hills (find a hilly route and run slightly faster than easy pace)
Week 7	Rest day	6 miles easy	8 miles with hills (find a hilly route and run slightly faster than easy pace) OR find a hill with 10 percent grade and do this workout: 2 miles easy 24 x 20-second sprints uphill with jog-down recovery 2 miles easy
Week 8	Rest day	9 miles speed workout: Yasso 800s 2 miles easy 6 x 800 meters at 10K pace with 400-meter recovery between 2 miles easy	6 miles easy
Week 9	6 miles easy	Rest day	7 miles easy
Week 10	4 miles easy	4 miles with fartlek: 1 mile easy 2 miles of 1 minute at 5K effort/1 minute easy 1 mile easy	Rest day

Rest day = Either take off or do 30 to 60 minutes of nonimpact or low-impact aerobic activity, such as cycling, elliptical training, or swimming.

	THURSDAY	FRIDAY	SATURDAY	SUNDAY
	6 miles easy	8 miles pace workout: 2 miles easy 4 miles at half-marathon pace 2 miles easy	5 miles easy	15 miles easy
	7 miles easy	Rest day	7 miles easy	10 miles with pace work: 2 miles easy 6 miles at half-marathon pace 2 miles easy
	8 miles with pace work: 2 miles easy 5 miles at half-marathon pace 1 mile easy	Rest day	6 miles easy	13 miles easy
	8 miles w/pace work: 3 miles easy 4 miles at half-marathon pace 1 mile easy	Rest day	6 miles easy	8 miles easy
	4 miles easy	Rest day	20 minutes easy + 4 x 20-second strides	Race day

RACING THE HALF MARATHON

For beginners, the goal is to cover the distance and finish happy, healthy, and strong. You don't need to warm up for this distance. Use the beginning miles to ease in. Begin conservatively—the first 6 miles should feel easy. Then hang on to that effort through the second half. Again, the only goal is to finish. Don't worry about your time.

For experienced runners, depending on your goals for the day and the kind of course you'll be racing on, you can approach the half marathon in several different ways.

THE WARMUP. As with any race, it's important to arrive with plenty of time to spare. Even though the miles are longer, it's still beneficial to warm up before you enter your corral. Experienced runners should jog for about 15 minutes and fit in 6 x 20-second strides as close to race time as possible. If newer runners choose to warm up, jog very easily for 10 minutes or briskly walk for 10 minutes and do 4 x 20-second strides. Begin that jog or brisk walk about 30 to 45 minutes before the race starts.

THE BEGINNING. As the race distance extends, attention to your pace at the beginning becomes more critical. The biggest mistake you can make in the half marathon (or marathon) is to start too fast. Pretend that your energy is being stored in a bank. Once you spend it, just like your money, it's gone. You can't get it back. So don't splurge in the first half. Physiologically you need to run slightly slower than your threshold (half-marathon) pace for as long as possible. That means the opening miles should be about 10 seconds slower than your goal pace.

THE MIDDLE MILES. When we think of "halfway" of the half marathon, we're tempted to place it, mathematically, at mile 6.5 or so. Logically that makes sense. But physiologically and psychologically, it's better to think of halfway as mile 10. You want the beginning to feel easy, then the middle to feel manageable. So gradually and slightly increase your pace beginning around mile six and keep it hard but sustainable until mile 10.

THE END. Your effort to sustain the pace is going to feel harder with about 5K to go, but thankfully you've prepared for this in your training, so call on all those hard workouts that you completed successfully. You're prepared for this. It is the time to start competing with the people around you. Start focusing on those just ahead and try to reel them in. Save a final gear for the last mile or so, and use it.

Chapter 6

Training for and Racing Marathons

Choosing and preparing for a marathon, race strategies, and key workouts

It wasn't long after I raced that very first 10K that I started becoming curious about the marathon distance. I was encouraged by my brother George's faith in me and inspired when he said he thought I had an ability to do well. I began to buckle down, and I decided to sign up for the *Prevention* Marathon in Bethlehem, Pennsylvania, the following year. I finished in 3:13 and not more than 2 months later decided to take another stab at 26.2 miles on Long Island in New York, where I clocked a 3:06.

That's the lure of the marathon—you have to study it and

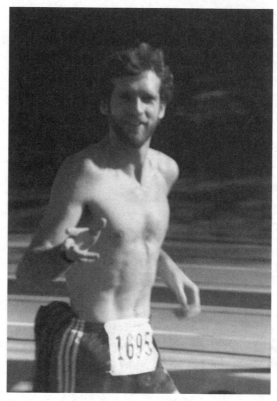

Cool as a cucumber at his second marathon ever, Bart cruises to a 3:06 finish on Long Island in New York.

experience it to get better at it. It's almost addictive in some ways. There always seem to be areas to improve, to have a better race strategy, to change training for next time, which is what keeps so many of us coming back to it. I was 25 years old at the time and decided that qualifying for the Boston Marathon would be my next goal, which meant I had to run a 2:50 or faster, which was then the qualifier for men in the 19 to 39 age bracket. I lifted weights, I added 20-mile long runs on Sundays, and I upped my mileage to 90 miles per week. I was serious. And by the fall of 1981, I was ready to toe the line at the Philadelphia marathon.

That day I knew I'd cut it close. And I did. I could see the finish line when the clock read 2:49:20. My father was waiting at the end, and I could also spot him in the crowd. All the sensations that so many others have been through on the quest for the Boston qualifier started to manifest: agony, numbness, burning, and the intense desire to vomit. I made it in 2:50:59—just a second to spare. With no chip timing in the 1980s, your time was exactly what the race clock said, and you had to wait a few weeks to receive an official time written on a postcard and mailed by the race. Most runners can't imagine not having an instant result, much less the agony of a gun time with thousands of people now lining up at the starts of races everywhere. Nevertheless, I was going to Boston, and I couldn't have been more pleased.

Men 40 and older had to clock 3:10 in those days to make it to Beantown. There was only one Boston qualifying time for women of all ages then, which was 3:20. If somebody didn't finish Boston faster than 3:35, they weren't recorded as a finisher in the results book. It was cutthroat stuff, to say the least. Of course, not as many people dared to run the distance back then, so times were naturally faster than after people of all abilities started running 26.2 miles with goals of finishing or checking off bucket-list items. The marathon is more welcoming to everybody now.

Nonetheless, getting that qualifying time is what so many recreational runners dream about achieving. While the professionals in this sport plan to peak in 4-year cycles, hoping to make it to the Olympic Trials and, ultimately, the Olympics, we mere mortals have this ongoing fascination and hope of racing Boston. For some, it's an easily attainable goal. For others, it requires years of training and many attempts to get there. Today, even running the qualifying time sometimes doesn't automatically mean you'll gain entry into the race—you have to run minutes faster than that to get your shot at registering.

But Boston, though the oldest and most prestigious marathon in the country, isn't the only one worthy of our respect and attention, of course—about 1,100 of them are held each year in the United States alone. I think I've probably run or attended nearly all of them . . . at least it seems like it. Some of my most vivid memories of my running career come from the many 26.2-mile races I've finished. For many years I focused on how fast I could get. And I got pretty fast, with a lifetime personal best of 2:40. As I got older and encountered more health issues, like my Lyme disease, I realized there was more to it than that: Appreciating the community, the scenery, and the spirit of this distance, not to mention the sense of accomplishment that comes from preparing for and finishing it, are all reasons we're drawn to the marathon time and again.

RACING THE NEW YORK CITY MARATHON

I find that each 26.2-mile race has its own niche and draw. The New York City Marathon just feels like the Olympics for the average runner. The run through the five boroughs, each with its own ethnic flair; the international presence of runners from around the world; the unbelievable spectator support—all of it conspires to make it an incredibly special event for everybody. It's the melting pot of running, with participants from 120 different countries. Then, as you progress through all parts of the city—Staten Island, Brooklyn, Queens, the Bronx, and Manhattan—it's obvious what neighborhood you're in from the storefronts and the people cheering out on the streets.

My favorite part of the course is between miles 15 and 16, when you're going over the Queensboro Bridge. With no spectators or traffic on the bridge, it's silent except for the pitter-pattering of feet. It's hard to imagine being in the middle of such a massive, bustling city and finding such a peaceful, quiet place. It's serenity with an incredible view. Many runners who have never raced the New York

City Marathon remark that that stretch of the course is so unexpected in an otherwise boisterous event.

Those who have never done this race before are equally shocked at what awaits immediately after the Queensboro Bridge. They have no idea what's going to hit them at mile 16.5, when they descend onto First Avenue in Manhattan. All of a sudden you're jolted out of that quiet time with this wall of people absolutely screaming their support at you. I don't know of anything else quite like it—except perhaps the women cheering at Wellesley College at the Boston Marathon. It's deafening and exciting, and it's probably the reason so many people end up running too fast up First Avenue (but more on that later). It's like you've hit a home run at game seven of the World Series at the bottom of the ninth inning. It's loud and exhilarating.

The New York City Marathon is a must-do at least once for any marathoner. But it's not an easy race to run, so here are my insider tips for racing in the Big Apple.

➤ CONSERVING YOUR ENERGY IN NEW YORK IS CRITICAL.

The logistics, the pace of city life, the sheer number of activities going on in the days leading up to the race can drain you. While you want to savor your experience, you'll also want to make sure you're not exhausting yourself before marathon day. Even the expo is big, and you could spend hours walking around it. Before you arrive in New York, plot out your itinerary and make sure you're not overdoing it. You'll want some downtime to put your feet up, relax, and rest.

➤ PREPARE FOR YOUR MORNING AT FORT WADSWORTH.

Race day in New York is equally taxing, and not just because of your 26.2-mile adventure back to Central Park. In 2016 the marathon had almost 51,400 finishers—making it the largest one in the world. Somehow, all those people have to make it out to

Staten Island, which means most of them will take a ferry from lower Manhattan in the wee hours of the morning. After you get there, you'll be in the athlete village, out in the elements, for a few hours before your wave is called to the corrals on the Verrazano Bridge. That means you need to preplan your transportation and the clothing, blankets, and additional food you'll want to stay warm and dry and fed, plus any supplies you'll need throughout the race. While you may be waking up at 4 a.m., it will still be a long time until you begin your race. Planning ahead is critical. I also recommend bringing some magazines, a newspaper, or a deck of cards to pass the time.

➤ **THE COURSE IS NOT EASY.** The tour of the five boroughs is scenic, the crowd support is second to none, and the camaraderie of fellow runners is constant. But the course is challenging. The five bridges interspersed throughout the 26.2 miles are all hills as you go up and over them. First Avenue is slightly uphill. Fifth Avenue, when you hit Manhattan, is gradually uphill. The final miles in Central Park and 59th Street are . . . you guessed it . . . hilly. All of these are deceptive inclines. You wouldn't necessarily find any of them difficult taken individually on a shorter run. Combine them over 26 miles, however, and your legs will feel them.

➤ **FIRST AVENUE IS A TRAP.** When you come off the Queensboro Bridge to your hero's welcome on First Avenue, you will start moving faster, not only because thousands of people are screaming at you, but because all the other runners around you have the same natural reaction at the same time—to speed up. Don't fall for it. It's way too early to hit the gas pedal. Enjoy the energy of the crowd, but don't feed too much off it. The people who go too fast on First Avenue are the ones struggling mightily in the Bronx.

➤ **ENJOY THE FINAL 200 METERS.** Very few finish lines have the history and emotional charge as the one at Tavern on the Green in Central Park. Everybody is greeted like a rock star. Look around, take it in, raise your hands up in the air, and smile. It's just one of those experiences that every runner should cherish. And then get ready for the longest marathon cooldown in the country. You'll be walking for a while before you exit the park onto Central Park West to find your loved ones in the expansive family-reunion area. But don't worry—your celebrity status is just beginning. Wear that finisher medal everywhere you go and you'll likely find yourself waved through the subway turnstiles and the first in line for a cab. It's your day in New York City and nobody lets you forget that, so celebrate it.

RACING THE BOSTON MARATHON

My first Boston Marathon came in 1982, which most running fans remember as the "Duel in the Sun" between Alberto Salazar and Dick Beardsley, who battled it out until the final 50 yards of the race, under clear skies, bright sun, and near-70 degrees. Salazar won in 2:08:51, a course record at the time and also notable in that era that two men had dipped under 2:09. Beardsley finished just 3 seconds later. It was a thrilling time to be in Boston, and I took full advantage of my debut at the prestigious event.

The biggest lesson I learned the first time I ran the Boston Marathon is that before you go, you have to decide how you plan to shape the experience. If you've never been to this event before, it's hard to predict how you'll react to it. The tradition, the pomp and circumstance, and the heightened sense of importance and pride throughout the city are palpable. You don't realize how much you're absorbing all of that in the excitement of finally being part of it.

Wherever you go, you're treated like a running superhero, and most of us have never experienced that before—by the time you're boarding the bus to Hopkinton on Marathon Monday, you are already a little spent, to be honest.

In 1982 I got caught up in the hoopla. I went to every seminar, headed to Bill Rodgers's running store ("Boston Billy" had won the marathon four times), and then decided to tour the Freedom Trail, visit the aquarium, and go to Cheers (the bar). They were all things I wanted to do, but doing them all in the days before running 26.2 miles didn't set me up for my greatest race. Although I felt like I was in 2:45 shape, I barely broke 3:00. For some runners, that's okay. The goal was to qualify for Boston, but the race itself is a form of celebration, and having fun is the primary purpose. It's just important to decide that before you arrive and psychologically accept it during

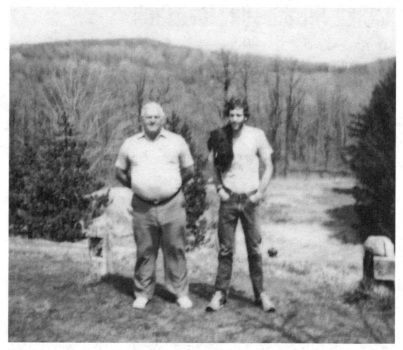

Bart shared his Boston Marathon weekend experience with is father (left).

the race to avoid feelings of failure or defeat on Boylston Street.

No matter what you decide to make your priority, save some time to do an important rite of passage before race day, when the street is finally shut down to traffic (usually on Sunday). Go down to the finish line and take pictures. Gaze down the famed Boylston Street and think about what it will be like to make the left-hand turn for the final stretch, with thousands of people cheering you on like you're in first place. So many runners dream of doing what you're about to do—you've probably dreamed a lot about it, too. You've made it, so give yourself a few moments to relish it while you take in running's most famed finish line.

My first Boston Marathon was my fourth marathon. I had a good formula for training, beginning around January 1. The hills of Boston are legendary, of course, so after I completed my typical base training, I focused on hill training, then included some speed sessions. As you may have noticed, I've been a proponent of including hilly runs in all of my training, but for Boston I tried to simulate when the hills came on the course, after 14 miles. I wanted to prepare for the Newton hills around mile 16, ending with Heartbreak Hill just before 21 miles.

During the race I realized what most rookies realize at their first Boston: I hadn't done enough downhill running in training. My quads were toast by the time I entered Newton. The descents in the first half of the race had left their mark. It's rare to leave your house for a training run and go downhill for 2 miles, but that's essentially the Boston Marathon course.

The following year, I ran 19 minutes faster at Boston than my first time there. Perhaps it was because we had cooler weather in 1983, but I suspect it had more to do with understanding the course a little better. I implemented downhill sections into the beginning of my long runs. It's important to learn how to handle those early descents if you want to run a good Boston Marathon.

Bart's Boston Workout: How to Callous Your Quads

On Marathon Monday the key to a happy, successful race is a pair of quads that can sustain a lot of downhill. Much is made of Heartbreak Hill, but honestly, it's a small concern in comparison to the damage from the first few downhill sections that can cause a lot of pain later in the race if you haven't prepped your body for the pounding.

I came up with a key workout that will help you prepare your quads for a beating in Boston. Do this 3 weeks before race day and schedule it for a day when the long run is behind you and you don't have any other critical workouts coming in the days ahead.

1. Warm up 2 miles easy, ending at the top of a hill that will take you 1 to 2 minutes to run down at a fast pace. It should be steep, but it should still allow you to remain controlled at a decent pace.

2. Run down the hill fast, around 5K pace, 6 to 10 times, jogging back up between repeats.

3. Cool down 2 miles easy.

Warning: This workout isn't going to feel difficult like most do. You're not going to feel taxed like a typical speed day. But if you did it right, you're going to wake up with sore quads. If you do, the mission is accomplished. You want to induce some short-term muscle damage that hurts for a couple of days. Run easy until the soreness goes away, about 3 days.

You only need one intense downhill session to have the protective effect for race day that will reduce the chances of your quads hurting on Marathon Monday. You still need to respect the distance, though. Take those opening hills easy and you'll thank yourself profusely around mile 18.

Let's Talk about the Weather

As I mentioned, the first year I ran on Marathon Monday it was sunny and warm. There's very little shade on the course (most people claim there's exactly none), and it's a shock to the system when you've done the bulk of your training during the winter months. But the weather in Boston is unpredictable. One year it's hot, the next year there's a nor'easter. There have been significant tailwinds and crazy headwinds. You just never know what you're going to get during the spring in New England, which is part of what makes the Boston Marathon the event that it is.

My advice is to pack gear for all seasons—and that's the case for nearly all marathons, not just Boston. If it's going to be a bright, sunny day with little cloud cover, you'll run slower because your skin temperature will increase and your ability to keep cool will diminish. Less blood goes to your working muscles when it's being sent to your skin. The sun will also hamper hydration, of course. As you sweat more, you'll lose more fluids.

How can you plan ahead? Well, that day in 1982 I was completely unprepared to face the conditions. I had done most of my training at 6 a.m. before work and 6 p.m. after work. It was dark outside. I never saw the sun. This was also back in the days when Boston started at noon.

Now it begins earlier, but only by about 2 hours, so most people will still be running during the midday hours.

If I had to do it over for my first Boston, I probably would have switched much of my training to lunchtime, so I could at least gain some exposure to the warmer, sunnier parts of the day. I certainly would have scheduled many more of my weekend long runs for the late morning, too. While it's unorthodox for most runners not to get up and at 'em first thing on a Sunday morning, you can practice a few times when the forecast might call for clear, warmer weather. That way you can also practice fueling and hydration prerace plans for race day, when you'll also begin running at a later hour than usual.

If all else fails, try doing some of your Boston Marathon training on the treadmill. I know many people hate the thought of staying indoors, but it provides a warmer climate that might allow greater adaptation to those conditions should they arise on Marathon Monday. But then again, you never know what Mother Nature has in store on Patriots' Day in Massachusetts, so your best bet is to not worry too much about the weather and always adapt your race plan and goals to whatever you're facing that day.

Race Morning in Hopkinton

The logistics and early morning rituals for Boston runners are similar to those of the New York City Marathon. An early-morning wake-up call, followed by a long ride on a big yellow school bus to Hopkinton, followed by a few hours of waiting outdoors in the athlete village before you're finally called to your wave and corral. Again, it takes some preparation and mental capacity to factor it all into your marathon-day strategy.

Most paramount to success on race day is getting fueling and hydration right that morning. For many people, the formula has come down to waking up, eating a decent breakfast, beginning the continual sips of water and sports drink, and maybe having that cup of coffee you normally have each day. Whatever it is, it should be what you've practiced on long-run days during training.

But that breakfast isn't the only one you should eat that day. Before race day, pack a second breakfast that you'll eat about 90 minutes or so before the race. It can be smaller than your first meal, but easily digestible to top off your glycogen stores so you're starting with a full tank. If possible, try the whole routine on one of your final long runs before Marathon Monday.

When I ran Boston I didn't know to do any of this, nor did I fuel up before or during my long runs. We just didn't do that back then. So on race day I didn't eat breakfast either, because I was afraid of throwing up or having to make a bathroom stop during the race. Also, they passed out salt tablets on the starting line and told us to swallow them. I had never done that before. Can you imagine? It probably doesn't need to be said, but never try anything new on race day. So you can predict what happens when your race starts at noon and you haven't had a morsel to eat all day, with 26.2 miles ahead of you. It's crazy to even think that's how we raced back then, but we did.

In the years after that I trained my gut to accept some toast before long runs. You can use your weeks of preparation to train your gut, too. Figure out when you should consume your breakfast, what your GI system will accept, and how you feel during your run. Adjust and experiment until you discover the right formula for you. You want to process what you've eaten before you get to the starting line. Pro tip: There are plenty of porta-potties in the athlete village, but there are usually also a bunch closer to the starting line with shorter lines because nobody realizes they're available.

And just like New York, you'll want to take blankets, extra throw-away clothing, and something relaxing to pass the time, like cards or reading material. Find a spot to sit and relax; resist the temptation to walk around. Don't forget to eat that second light breakfast and try to stay out of the sun if you can—or out of the snow, sleet, hail, or torrential rain. (Who knows? Like I said—spring in New England is for hardy souls.) Remember to focus only on things you can control. The weather is not one of them.

Handling the Boston Marathon Course

Contrary to popular belief, you can run a smart race in Boston. I'm sure of it. You can also run a negative split (cover the second half faster than the first) if you play your cards right. So what if the first 13.1 miles are riddled with downhill miles and the second have all the uphill? If you look at the professional runners' times, many of the best of them over history have run faster during the second

13.1 miles. The last 5 miles can be fast if your quads are causing you issues (if they are, you'll be cursing every downhill you encounter). If you have something left to pick up the pace, it will fuel your mental game, too.

My best race in Boston was in 1984 when I finished in 2:41—a day that brought cold temperatures and a nasty headwind. I adjusted my goals before I went to the starting line, knowing that the weather conditions probably weren't conducive to running my fastest. It was a rare display of wisdom and restraint—we were all kind of knuckleheads back then and too stubborn for our own good, so I'll give myself some credit in this scenario.

The thing is, I think most smart runners account for the many variables that Boston presents and decide that it isn't a PR course. Few people say that their best marathon time was set in Boston, although it can happen. Ryan Hall, the two-time Olympic marathoner who retired from competitive running in 2016, ran his fastest 26.2 miles there in 2011, which was a year that showcased a pretty hefty tailwind. He cruised in for a 2:04:58. The overall course is net downhill, but as I've said, the route's design is brutal on the body.

A few pieces of advice:

➤ **YOU'RE RUNNING WITH YOUR PEERS.** You'll be assigned to a corral with runners who qualified with about the same time you did. That means most of them are exactly your ability level. That makes it easy to collectively work together, if you choose. Some probably have similar goals for the day that you do. Introduce yourself and find some new running buddies—you can keep each other in check through those critical early miles. If you hang on to each other through the Newton Hills, you can also take turns helping the group pick up the pace. Teamwork makes the dream work, of course.

➤ **THE STREETS ARE NARROW EARLY ON.** You begin in the quaint town of Hopkinton on a normal two-lane road, with thousands of your best friends. Within only a few steps off the line, you're heading downhill. It's like jumping off a cliff. Well, not really, but pay attention to your pace and don't get caught up with the folks who are going way too fast just because you're sort of packed in like sardines at that early stage.

➤ **FOCUS ON AN EVEN PACE IN THE FIRST HALF.** The beginning 13.1 miles feel easy. You'll probably look down at your watch and see that your splits are too fast, but you're feeling so good you won't care. You will care a lot more about this later if you keep it up. Remind yourself that soon you won't be feeling that well. If you get carried away and blitz your halfway split, chances are your quads are about to punch you back in the later miles. You don't want to stumble down Boylston Street—you want to look like the champion you are. Tell yourself to cool it.

➤ **FORGET ABOUT PACE THROUGH NEWTON.** When you hit the famous "Newton Hills" from miles 16 to 21, don't look at your watch. Try to keep an even effort through this part instead of an even pace. If you begin breathing harder than you were, back off a little bit. That's why I don't run with music. I want to be in tune with my body's signals. I don't suggest anybody use the phrase "attack the hills." That's just asking for trouble because the hills always win. It's not a fair fight, especially at the marathon distance. Just cruise up them at an even effort and don't look down at your watch.

➤ **AT THE TOP OF HEARTBREAK HILL, GO FOR IT.** You're facing a lot of downhill again at this point, so if you conserved enough energy, you should have something in the tank to let loose a little bit. Turn the legs over and don't be afraid to switch gears. You have nothing to lose.

(continued on page 108)

A Few of My Other Favorite Marathons

It's so difficult to select just a couple of the best 26.2 miles to talk about because I truly have a soft spot for so many of them. Here are a few more that have a place in my heart.

Big Sur Marathon: Everybody always says this one is so hard, but remember that the course offers more downhill than uphill. It does, though, predominantly have a headwind. Some years it's more of a factor than others. All

you have to do is train on hills during your long runs and you can do well here. What Big Sur is really about is the natural beauty running along the Pacific Ocean. The views are truly breathtaking. It's the only time they close California State Route 1 for a sporting event, which makes it special.

I was interviewed by the local newspaper after I ran it several years ago. The reporter looked me right in the eye and said,

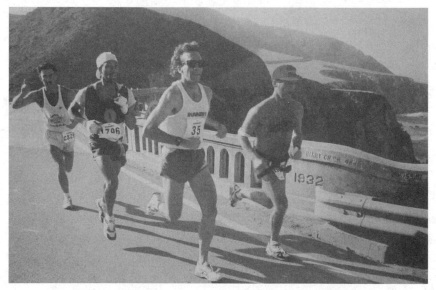

Running along the Pacific Ocean again, this time in the early days of the Big Sur Marathon.

"What did you think?" and I told her, "If I was told I could only do one marathon in my life, this would be the race." It's the prettiest stretch of road I've ever been on in the United States.

Catalina Island Marathon: All the runners stay in this little town, Avalon. The morning of the race, 1,200 runners get on a big catamaran that takes you to the other side of the island, called Two Harbors. It is a point-to-point course across the island. You start on a grass runway where private planes take off and land, then turn right, then go 3 miles uphill on single-track trail. You go back down to sea level, then climb again; around the 23-mile mark you look down and see the finish line. It's all downhill back into Avalon. I'm just drawn to untouched natural habitats. It's gorgeous and disconnected from the world. You're isolated 26 miles out in the ocean. I love trails and mountains, so this one is right up my alley. If you go, try to prepare on some single track if you have access, though the terrain is not that technical, so any-

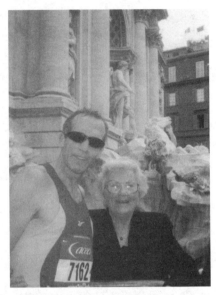

Bart stops for a hug from his mom during the Rome Marathon.

body will be fine on the course. It's not a race to go by time—instead of splits, just go by feel.

Rome Marathon: I can't think of another race that showcases the city's history and attractions better than this one. You run on a lot of cobblestone, which can be a little taxing, but it's not as bad as you may imagine. And don't forget you're in Europe. The

(continued)

course is marked in kilometers, not miles. Although the course has changed over the years, it still takes you by some of the most amazing sites. When I ran in 2001, we began in the shadow of the Colosseum, then ran along the Tiber River and past the Trevi Fountain, St. Peter's Basilica, the Spanish Steps, and Piazza Navona. The last 3 miles of the race were on the Appian Way, which conjures images of Roman soldiers in 300 BC or thereabouts. But it's also where Abebe Bikila won the 1960 Olympic marathon, coming through in the dark with lit torches lining the street, 24 years after Mussolini had conquered his homeland of Ethiopia. He was the first African to win an Olympic medal—and he did it barefoot because his shoes didn't fit correctly. The actual finish line of the race was at the Arco di Costantino. I don't think you can find a finish line better than that.

My mom came to watch the Rome Marathon the year I ran, and I stopped to give her a hug and take a photo with her at the Trevi Fountain along the way. I didn't know it at the time, but after she passed away, that picture captured my all-time favorite running moment. I'll always cherish it.

Chicago Marathon: Whatever your pace is, get on it at the beginning and you'll just become a metronome until the finish. There's not an inkling of an incline until mile 25.9, then there's a short climb up to the finish line. I led the 3-hour pace group in 1997, and it was so easy to stay right on that pace because there's just no change in elevation. You have to be ready for crowds. Every neighborhood has droves of people out cheering. The finish in Grant Park is packed, too. The advantage of

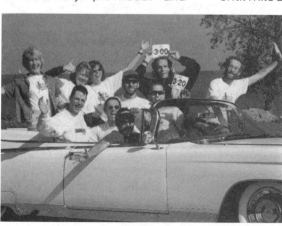

The Runner's World *pacers are ready to hit the streets of Chicago in 1997.*

Chicago compared to many big city marathons is that the logistics are easier. The start and finish are close together and within walking distance to many hotels, so it's convenient. You eliminate the transportation and long waiting periods before the race, which helps you save a lot of energy. For those who like to run even splits, this is your race. If you want to run fast at a big-city marathon in the United States, Chicago is the place to go.

Marine Corps Marathon: This one is vital in the big picture. Without the people who put on the Marine Corps Marathon, we would not have the freedom to run all these other races. It's an emotional course because you see images such as Arlington Cemetery, Iwo Jima Memorial, and mile 10.5, which is dedicated to fallen servicemen and -women. Gold Star families and friends from Wear Blue: Run to Remember line the street with American flags and photos of their fallen family members in a touching tribute. I find it to be the most emotional mile of any race I've ever done.

And, of course, on top of those iconic places, there are more. You also go past the National Mall, the Pentagon, and the Washington Monument. There is one bugger of a hill at the finish line. It's the steepest, shortest finish line in all of marathons, I think, but it ends at the Iwo Jima Memorial, which is the point. Save a little something to get yourself up that incline. Nobody wants to walk over a marathon finish line no matter where it is, but especially in front of a bunch of Marines.

To see all the military presence out on the course is moving. I ran this race in 2001, 5 weeks after 9/11. I was leading a pace group around 3 hours. In the early miles I've always found runners to be a bit boisterous because it feels easy at that point. I remember a lot of banter going on, and then we came up toward the Pentagon. As we got closer, we could see the gaping hole in the building where the plane crashed just weeks earlier. The group was suddenly silent. You could hear a pin drop. The only sounds were our breathing and our footsteps. Nobody knew what to say—at that point in American history we had so few words for what had happened. But everybody in my group was locked in on the Pentagon. Back then, the course got really close to the building. It's an image I will never forget.

➤ **ABSORB THE CROWD'S ENERGY.** The spectators in Boston are the most educated marathon fans you'll find. They line the course from start to finish and they are extremely loud. You might lose your hearing when you hit halfway and run past the Wellesley College women. It's deafening—the decibel level is something I can't find the words to adequately describe. You're not going to avoid frenzy, so embrace it and use it to your advantage during the low points. But don't let the enthusiasm get the best of you, propelling you to unsustainable paces. Keep a level head. It's up to you if you accept the beer offerings when you run through the Boston College crowd.

TRAINING FOR A MARATHON

Everybody has their own take on what the "best" marathon training program is, and perhaps all of them are right. My take is that the right plan is the one that works for you.

When you train for marathons, you have to pay a lot of attention to your lifestyle. The demands of your job, family, friends, and other circumstances have to be taken into account. Most marathon training plans call for a dedicated 16 to 20 weeks of commitment. That's not a short amount of time to dedicate to a hobby, so be sure that not only are you on board, but those who support you and depend on you are also signed off on it. Chances are you're going to miss a few events or let the grass grow a little too long before it's all said and done.

For first-time marathoners, it's best to have at least 6 months of consistent running under your belt before you target 26.2 miles. You should try a 5K, 10K, and half marathon first and feel comfortable running 4 days a week. Again, don't rush this process for the sake of checking off a bucket-list item. If you do this right and follow a gradual progression toward this admirable goal, you'll enjoy the process and the experience a lot more. You'll also reduce your chances of burnout and injury. All of this adds up to a continued love of running, and that's what we should all want.

The most important part of marathon training for me has always been the weekly long run. While many people like to include some sort of marathon pace into these runs, I've always done better to keep them at the slower, conversational pace and practice more speed during midweek runs. It's okay to go 1 minute per mile slower than your goal marathon pace when you're going long—and for newer runners, just keep it easy and sustainable. My longest runs during my buildup generally top out at 20 miles. For beginners, it's essential to understand that you do not need to cover a full 26 miles in your training to be able to finish on race day. You just need to stay consistent in your weekly training and build to about 18 to 20 miles for a long run.

Again, it's critical to think about recovery, fueling, and nutrition as you build up your mileage. Hopefully you started practicing good habits like getting enough sleep, eating whole foods, and drinking lots of water while you built up for the half marathon (for more information on recovery and fueling, see Chapter 5). These strategies are more amplified now that the volume of miles you're logging is increasing.

Beginner Marathon Training Plan

(Assumes a base of 25 miles per week)

	MONDAY	TUESDAY	WEDNESDAY
Week 1	4 miles easy	Rest day	4 miles easy
Week 2	4 miles easy	Rest day	3 miles easy
Week 3	Rest day	3 miles easy	4 miles easy + 4 x 20-second strides
Week 4	Rest day	4 miles easy	3 miles easy + 4 x 20-second strides
Week 5	3 miles easy	Rest day	4 miles fartlek: 2 miles easy 2 miles with 2 minutes on/2 minutes off
Week 6	3 miles easy	Rest day	5 miles easy
Week 7	Rest day	3 miles easy	4 miles fartlek: 1 mile easy 2 miles with 3 minutes on/1 minute off 1 mile easy
Week 8	Rest day	4 miles easy	5 miles easy + 4 x 20-second strides
Week 9	Rest day	4 miles easy	5 miles fartlek: 2 miles easy 2 miles with 4 minutes on/1 minute off 1 mile easy
Week 10	4 miles easy	Rest day	6 miles easy

THURSDAY	FRIDAY	SATURDAY	SUNDAY
Rest day	6 miles easy	Rest day	6 miles easy
4 miles easy	Rest day	4 miles easy	8 miles easy
3 miles easy	Rest day	3 miles easy	10 miles easy
4 miles easy	Rest day	3 miles easy	11 miles easy
Rest day	5 miles easy	Rest day	12 miles easy
4 miles easy + 4 x 20-second strides	Rest day	3 miles easy	10 miles easy
3 miles easy	Rest day	4 miles easy	14 miles easy
Rest day	4 miles easy	4 miles easy	15 miles easy
5 miles easy	Rest day	3 miles easy	12 miles easy
5 miles easy + 6 x 20-second strides	3 miles easy	Rest day	16 miles

(continued)

Beginner Marathon Training Plan *(cont.)*

	MONDAY	TUESDAY	WEDNESDAY	
Week 11	4 miles easy	Rest day	6 miles fartlek: 3 miles easy 2 miles with 5 minutes on/2 minutes off 1 mile easy	
Week 12	3 miles easy	Rest day	6 miles easy	
Week 13	3 miles easy	Rest day	6 miles fartlek: 2 miles easy 3 miles with 5 minutes on/2 minutes off 1 mile easy	
Week 14	3 miles easy	Rest day	7 miles easy	
Week 15	Rest day	6 miles easy	4 miles fartlek: 2 miles easy 2 miles with 3 minutes on/1 minute off	
Week 16	3 miles easy	Rest day	4 miles easy + 4 x 20-second strides	

Easy = Pace that you can sustain for long periods of time. You could carry on a conversation without any problem at this pace.

Strides = Do these on a flat surface, gradually accelerating to about 90 percent effort. Take full recovery before starting the next one.

THURSDAY	FRIDAY	SATURDAY	SUNDAY
4 miles easy	4 miles easy	Rest day	18 miles
6 miles easy + 6 x 20-second strides	Rest day	4 miles easy	16 miles
4 miles easy	3 miles easy or cross-train 30 minutes	Rest day	20 miles
5 miles easy + 6 x 20-second strides	Rest day	5 miles easy	12 miles easy
4 miles easy	Rest day	4 miles easy	6 miles easy
3 miles easy	Rest day	20 minutes easy + 6 x 20-second strides	Race day

Rest day = Either take off or do 30 minutes of nonimpact or low-impact aerobic activity, such as cycling, elliptical training, or swimming.

Fartlek = For beginners, the "on" segments should be faster than easy pace but not sprints. Find a pace that is challenging but sustainable. "Off" segments should be easy pace.

Seasoned-Runner Marathon Training Plan

(Assumes previous marathon training experience and a base of 35 miles per week)

	MONDAY	TUESDAY	WEDNESDAY
Week 1	5 miles easy	6 miles easy	Rest day
Week 2	5 miles easy	6 miles easy	Rest day
Week 3	Rest day	4 miles easy	6 miles on hilly terrain
Week 4	Rest day	6 miles on a hilly route	7 miles easy
Week 5	Rest day	6 miles on a hilly route	6 miles easy

THURSDAY	FRIDAY	SATURDAY	SUNDAY
6 miles fartlek: 2-mile warmup 10 x 2 minutes at 10K effort/90 seconds easy 1-mile warmdown	Rest day	5 miles easy	8 miles easy
6 miles pace workout: 2 miles easy 2 miles at marathon pace 2 miles easy	Rest day	6 miles easy	10 miles easy
Rest day	8 miles pace workout: 2 miles easy 3 miles at marathon pace 3 miles easy	6 miles easy	12 miles easy
8 miles pace workout: 2 miles easy 4 miles at marathon pace 2 miles easy	Rest day	6 miles easy	12 miles easy
9 miles speed workout: 2 miles easy 5 miles at marathon pace 2 miles easy	Rest day	6 miles easy	13 miles easy

(continued)

Seasoned-Runner Marathon Training Plan (cont.)

	MONDAY	TUESDAY	WEDNESDAY
Week 6	4 miles easy	Rest day	7 miles speedwork: 2-mile warmup 4 x 800 meters at about 10K pace with 400-meter jog between 3-mile cooldown Yasso 800s
Week 7	Rest day	5 miles easy	8 miles with hills
Week 8	Rest day	9 miles speed workout: Yasso 800s 2 miles easy 6 x 800 meters at 10K pace with 400-meter recovery between 2 miles easy	6 miles easy
Week 9	6 miles easy	Rest day	7 miles with hill repeats (described in "Bart's Favorite Hill Workout," page 79)
Week 10	4 miles easy	Rest day	9 miles speed workout: 2 miles easy 6 x Yasso 800s 2 miles easy

THURSDAY	FRIDAY	SATURDAY	SUNDAY
6 miles easy	8 miles pace workouts: 2 miles easy 4 miles at half-marathon pace 2 miles easy	5 miles easy	14 miles easy
7 miles easy	9 miles with marathon pace: 2 miles easy 6 miles at marathon pace 1 mile easy	4 miles easy	15 miles easy
6 miles easy	8 miles with pace work: 1 mile easy 6 miles at marathon pace 1 mile easy	6 miles easy + 6 x 20-second strides	16 miles easy
7 miles easy	10 miles with pace work: 2 miles easy 7 miles at marathon pace 1 mile easy	6 miles easy + 6 x 20-second strides	12 miles easy
8 miles easy	10 miles with pace work: 1 mile easy 8 miles at marathon pace 1 mile easy	6 miles easy + 6 x 20-second strides	16 miles easy

(continued)

Seasoned-Runner Marathon Training Plan *(cont.)*

	MONDAY	TUESDAY	WEDNESDAY
Week 11	Rest day	6 miles easy	8 miles on a hilly route
Week 12	Rest day	6 miles easy	10 miles speed workout: 2 miles easy 8 x Yasso 800s 2 miles easy
Week 13	3 miles easy	Rest day	10 miles on a hilly course
Week 14	Rest day	7 miles easy	12 miles speed workout: 2 miles easy 10 x Yasso 800s 2 miles easy
Week 15	4 miles easy	Rest day	6 miles on hilly route
Week 16	Rest day	6 miles easy	4 miles easy

THURSDAY	FRIDAY	SATURDAY	SUNDAY
6 miles easy	10 miles with pace work: 1 mile easy 8 miles at marathon pace 1 mile	6 miles easy + 6 x 20-second strides	18 miles
6 miles easy	10 miles with pace work: 1 mile easy 8 miles at marathon pace 1 mile	3 miles easy + 6 x 20-second strides	20 miles
8 miles easy	12 miles with pace work: 2 miles easy 9 miles at marathon pace 1 mile easy	8 miles easy + 6 x 20-second strides	14 miles
6 miles easy	10 miles with pace work: 2 miles easy 7 miles at marathon pace 1 mile easy	Rest day	21 miles
6 miles easy	8 miles with pace work: 2 miles easy 5 miles at marathon pace 1 mile easy	6 miles easy + 6 x 20-second strides	10 miles easy
4 miles easy	Rest day	20 minutes easy + 6 x 20-second strides	Race day

Bart's Favorite Marathon Workout

Well, I think I'd be remiss if I didn't say that Yasso 800s are my favorite marathon workout. It isn't the only one I recommend, but it holds a special place in my heart (see Chapter 2 for the full story).

Yasso 800s

Workout: 10 x 800 meters completed in the time you are shooting for in the marathon, but in minutes and seconds. So if your goal is 3:30 in the marathon, you want to shoot for 3 minutes and 30 seconds per 800 meters. Usually that is somewhere between a 5K and 10K pace on the track. Take the same amount of rest between intervals that it took to run the 800 meters (so 3:30, using the same example) or simply jog 400 meters between each 800-meter interval. Warm up 20 minutes before the workout and cool down 20 minutes afterward.
When: Take your first crack at this workout about 2 months before your race. The first week, complete only 4 x 800 meters. Add one more 800 repeat per week until you are up to 10 x 800 meters. The last workout should be completed about 10 to 14 days before your marathon.

Marathon Pace Workout

It's the bread and butter of long-distance running. You can't skip it if you want to improve in the marathon.
Workout: Run easy for 15 minutes, ease into your goal marathon pace and sustain it for 45 to 60 minutes, run easy for 15 minutes.
When: You can do different variations of this run once a week throughout your training. Start at the low end of the length you're sustaining marathon pace and gradually build the time you're holding it every week.

RACING A MARATHON

Before you start training, you have to pick a marathon. When you make this decision, take several factors into account.

> **DO YOU WANT A BIG-CITY RACE? A MIDSIZE FIELD? OR SOMETHING LOCAL AND SMALL?** There are pros and cons to all of these options. It just depends on if you want to travel somewhere and be among thousands of others, which also means you'll have big crowds of supporters, or if you want to stay close to home and don't really care if you never see a soul along the way. And, of course, there are many options somewhere in between. My advice is to make your first marathon something that is logistically simple. It's enough that you're going to run 26.2 miles for the first time without adding a ferry ride or a 4-hour athlete village stay to the day. But, again, everybody is different—pick whatever is most motivating to you.

> **ARE YOU GOING FOR THE EXPERIENCE OR DO YOU WANT TO RUN A FAST RACE?** They aren't mutually exclusive goals, but some lesser-known races offer faster terrain. Do your research to figure out what plays to your strengths if a new PR is your aim.

> **WHAT TIME OF YEAR DO YOU PREFER?** If you pick a spring race, you'll likely train through some winter months in most areas of the country. If you pick a fall race, you'll deal with some hot summer running. Either time of year, of course, will throw some unpredictable conditions at runners. Think about other commitments in your life and when it might be most feasible to remain consistent in your training.

When you arrive at the starting line of the marathon, the best advice I can give you is to be confident in your preparation. Find a sense of peace knowing that you've done all the work. The race is merely a celebration of months of hard work. This is your reward for putting in all the miles, eating all the nutritious meals, and going to bed when everybody else is going out. You've earned this race and this day.

The biggest mistake anybody can make in racing a marathon is starting out too fast, of course. You have to start out conservatively and settle into your pace gradually. Typically, the beginning miles will be crowded, adrenaline-filled affairs. Don't waste your time weaving around people (just like every other race distance—do I sound like a broken record?). Just practice patience—you have hours ahead of you to find your groove. For those going for a specific time, averaging about 10 seconds faster or slower than your goal pace in the early miles is fine.

Fueling and hydrating are crucial in the marathon. You have to replace glycogen before you go into debt. If you don't fuel properly, you'll hit the inevitable "wall" right around 18 to 20 miles. Practice your fueling and hydration plan during your long runs leading up to the race. Plan ahead for when you'll take in calories and at what aid stations you'll grab water or sports drinks.

It's been said that in the marathon you run the first 20 miles with your head and the last 6.2 miles with your heart. To me, this means you want to stay as close to even splits as you can for the first 20 miles, then run by feel in the last 10K. You may slow a little bit in the later miles—many people do. The ultimate goal is to negative split, but it takes practice and skill to do this, as well as the perfect course that doesn't present challenges, such as hills, in the final miles. Up until mile 20 you want to keep yourself as controlled and relaxed as you can, almost zoning out at your goal pace. When you have 10K to go, you can't zone out anymore, though. You have to focus. Break it down into smaller parts if it helps you get through it—10 minutes at a time or 5K at a time, whatever works for you.

In an ideal world, you'd have something left in the final miles to pick up your pace. It takes a perfectly executed race plan to allow that to happen. If you feel like you can roll a little faster, go for it with 5K left. Hopefully you're well on your way to your strongest finish yet.

Chapter 7

Training for and Racing Ultramarathons

Choosing and preparing for an ultramarathon, race strategies, and key workouts

I will begin by telling you not to start running ultramarathons in the same fashion I did. I wouldn't advise my method to anybody.

That said, I'll fill you in on my initiation into ultras. Don't try this at home, kids.

It was 1989 and a group of us from *Runner's World* were at a trade show together in Atlanta. The shoe company Hi-Tec, which had become the sponsor of the Badwater, a 146-mile race in July through Death Valley and to the top of Mount Whitney, started talking to us

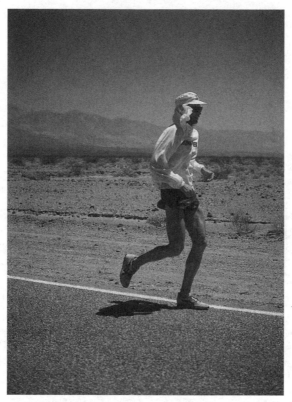

Bart's first ultramarathon was Badwater, one of the most challenging races on the planet.

about this little-known race (it no longer summits Whitney, so the course is now 135 miles). Back then people thought running 26.2 miles was extreme. Ultrarunning was by no means mainstream at the time—the Internet didn't exist, Instagram didn't exist, and therefore professional ultrarunners did not exist.

The shoe company wanted to bring more attention to Badwater, so George Hirsch, the publisher of *Runner's World* at the time, volunteered me to run it. Amby agreed that I was the only one among the group who would do such an outlandish thing. He was right.

Mind you, at the time I had never run more than 26.2 miles in one shot. Never mind that this race was 5.5 times longer than that, it was also held in 134-degree temperatures across the salty floor of Death Valley, up 14,496 feet above sea level to the top of Mount Whitney. The roads in between radiated 150-degree heat, while the wind and sandstorms whipped at your face. In 1989 the event was just 2 years old and boasted a whopping nine finishers. I wasn't fully convinced that I could add to that tally, but I was willing to give it a shot.

I didn't even like running in the heat, but nevertheless I gathered my crew—the poor souls who volunteered to support me through the race with positive reinforcement, food, hydration, and a kick in the pants if needed. Jane Serues, then *Runner's World*'s promotional director, and Bob "Wish" Wischnia, the deputy editor at the time, were on board. They dutifully met me every mile in an RV stocked with $300 worth of groceries and more water than any group of human beings could possibly consume, even a group traveling across such brutal territory. Either we were really off with our calculations or we didn't want to leave hydration to chance.

I knew that I had to just sustain an extremely slow pace. Back then I didn't realize that it was okay to walk at any point, though I did for a couple of brief stretches. People just didn't do that at the time—runners ran, no matter how slowly. I was convinced that if I walked very much, some god of running would strike me down and that would be the end of it. Around mile 45 the Hi-Tec reps dropped off Steve Flanagan. He was a sales director, 2:18 marathoner, and member of the US world cross-country team. Impressive credentials—though today he's better known as father of Shalane Flanagan, the country's top marathoner and 10,000-meter Olympic silver medalist in 2008. Anyway, I had to school Steve on how to pace an ultra. I was afraid he'd lure me into a faster pace, which would ruin me at this early juncture in the race. He did speed me up, but as we were heading up a mountain, Steve bailed after only a few miles—he said it was too hot. He headed back to his air-conditioned van and frosty beer.

I, however, forged on. We had to spend the night in Lone Pine because I hit that 125-mile mark just as it was about to get dark. I wouldn't be able to summit Mount Whitney and get back down before sunset. We headed back out 2 hours before the sun began to rise. When I hit the top, I was greeted by David Pompel, the race director, who said I had just completed the toughest footrace in the country—he could add one more to his list.

We'll never know where I placed because I never checked the results. It did launch me into notoriety in the running world, however. I was now known as Badwater Bart. Not only that, but race directors now realized that inviting me to their events would boost their promotional efforts. Consequently, I've been flooded with invitations ever since.

That was my introduction to ultramarathoning. Like I said—I don't recommend it.

What I did learn, however, is that I enjoyed the idea of running longer than 26.2 miles. An ultra distance is considered any race longer than a marathon. I also craved being in nature—the kind you can't find at road races—on trails, through the woods, up mountains. The appeal was there, and I wanted to pursue less extreme options than Badwater.

The progression into ultramarathons can, and should, be gradual. After you've done a marathon or two, try a 50K. When you feel comfortable at 50K, go for a 50 miler, then 100K, and maybe even eventually aim for a 100 miler. Just like all other distances, it's best to build up to these goals in a steady, consistent manner to avoid burnout, injury, and frustration.

I find that when the average runner is training for ultra distances for the first time (or *ever,* for many people), the aim isn't speed but covering the distance and finishing. This holds for ultras more than any other kind of race. Therefore, the training isn't so much speed

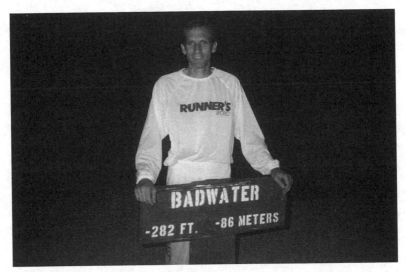

Bart prepares to embark on a 146-mile adventure.

focused, but it places a priority on the time you spend on your feet. You increase your long runs in minutes rather than miles and you implement back-to-back long runs on the weekends so your body can adapt to the fatigue and get stronger.

Training for an ultra of any distance is a big commitment. When you're not out there running, you'll likely feel tired. It's a big decision to sign up for a long race and one you should discuss with the people in your life because while you're preparing for it, you'll have to make some sacrifices that may impact your time with them or other responsibilities.

The return on your investment, however, is high. Many ultras take us to places you just can't reach other than to go there on foot. The camaraderie of the trail and ultrarunning communities is a huge draw. You'll find that it's close-knit, warm, and welcoming. And the accomplishment of completing a continuous 50K, 50 miles, or more is extraordinary.

COMRADES MARATHON:
THE MOST MEANINGFUL OF BART'S CAREER

It's the one that almost got away.

My entire running career, though fulfilling and fortunate in countless ways, always felt like something was missing that was important to me. I wanted more than anything to race the Comrades Marathon before it was all said and done.

The race, which is 56 miles (89K) between the cities of Durban and Pietermaritzburg in South Africa, had a spell over me. It was about to go down as my only regret in nearly 33 years of running because my Lyme disease, which I had been living with for more than a decade, was becoming debilitating.

When I climbed Mount Kilimanjaro in 1997 I had a serious bout of Lyme-related illness, which had been first diagnosed in 1990 after I ran the Lake Waramaug 50-miler in Connecticut. I made it all the way to Kibo Hut, the final camp, before summiting 6 miles later, when I had to call it quits. I woke up unable to see out of my right eye, which was paralyzed open—in fact, the right side of my face was paralyzed. I made it down to the bottom in 9 hours and ended up in a local hospital, where the staff was ill equipped and sent me to Nairobi. The paralysis started weakening my right lower extremities, too.

When I finally got home to Pennsylvania, I was diagnosed, again, with Lyme disease. And while I've had many quality years of running following that diagnosis, I've also endured a lot of physical pain and setbacks, which eventually led me to believe that I would never get to South Africa to run Comrades.

My fantasy began when I read about Comrades in the early 1980s. It's the oldest and largest ultramarathon in the world. The field is the size of a big-city marathon and the mountains make Heartbreak Hill look like a pancake. After I did my first 50 miler, which I finished in 6:11, I thought one day maybe I could finish in the top 50 at Comrades. But I felt like traveling to South Africa during Apartheid years was like supporting it, so I put that plan on hold.

By 1993 I had an opportunity to finally go, and my health prevented me from making the trip, which happened again years later. I had slowly started accepting that I might never make it, though it haunted me.

Why was Comrades so important? I wanted to experience this post-Apartheid change. If I had gone 30 years beforehand, younger and healthier, there would have been few black citizens in the race. Standing on that starting line, watching these black South African athletes ready to run sub–6-minute pace for 56 miles, singing their national anthem with tears running down their cheeks, I was so moved. It is what our sport is about—opening the opportunity for all people to get to the starting line and giving them a chance to see what they can do.

Though again not in good health, I decided to make it happen in

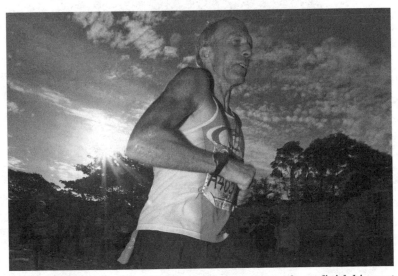

Struggling from mile 1, Bart powered through Comrades to finish his most meaningful race.

2010. I told myself if I could finish the marathon distances at all the events I was attending for work over the course of a few months, then I could finish Comrades. My training was essentially only doing one long run—a marathon—per weekend. My body couldn't handle any more than that.

I was in rough shape when we arrived in South Africa, but this time nothing was going to stop me from experiencing this race. My fear was that I would not make the cutoff time of 12 hours. The race officials lock the gate to the finish line at 12 hours and you aren't

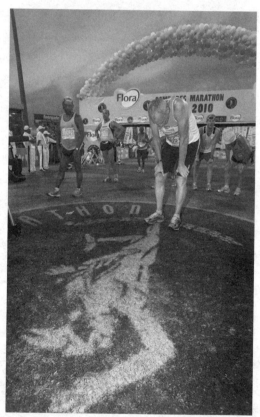

Bart didn't run as fast as he had hoped, but the finish line was sweet.

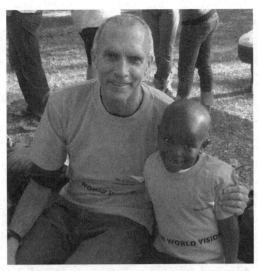

During the trip to South Africa, Team World Vision provided opportunities to meet local children.

allowed to cross it. After so many years and missed opportunities to be there, I couldn't let that happen. My joint pain radiated through my body, and swelling in my legs prevented me from having any kind of fluid stride—I limped from the first mile.

But I interacted with the South African people throughout the race. It was as magical as I had always imagined it would be. It was a "down" year—the race alternates directions, one uphill and the other down. As we ran through the villages where clean water and electricity are luxuries, the people came out in droves to support us. It carried me and put my personal worries into perspective.

Twenty-five miles in, I saw the 11-hour pace group ahead of me, about 1,000 people strong, and wanted so badly to catch it. I tried, but my body wouldn't let me. My legs just couldn't move any faster. Instead I pushed forward as best I could and actually was able to pick up my pace slightly. I knew I was still ahead of the cutoff time, though only by about a half hour.

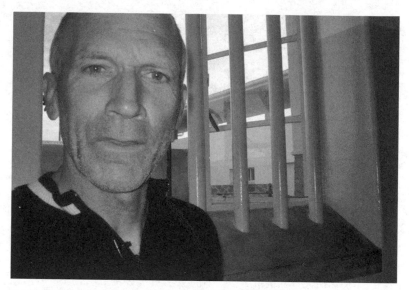

During the trip, Bart stopped to visit Nelson Mandela's jail cell.

I came across the finish line in 11:33:38. I had 27 minutes to spare, dragging my right leg to the end. It was like Boston, New York City, and the London marathons all rolled into one on the Fourth of July and Christmas Day. It's difficult to articulate why it was so meaningful. My brother George loved South Africa—he had always wanted to go there to compete in rugby, but he never had the chance. He died in 2003 of prostate cancer, having never fulfilled that wish. Part of me was there for him, and I thought a lot about him through the race.

After Comrades it took me more than 2 months to run another step. I was convinced it was my last race, and I was at peace with that. But as we all know now, it wasn't my final bow. Something about the running community continually lures me back in, despite the fact that I can no longer be competitive. Engaging with the people and hearing the kind of obstacles they've overcome to get to all of these races is nothing short of inspiring. It keeps me going (and going and going).

Racing Tips for Comrades

Like all ultramarathons, the biggest favor you can do for yourself is to make sure you've properly prepared not only for the distance, but for the terrain. Here are a few pointers.

➤ Investigate whether you will be running an "up" or a "down" year. A down year has about 7,000 feet of descent and 5,000 feet of ascent. An up year has the opposite. So either direction offers plenty of both kinds of hills. Either way, you'll want to implement the appropriate amount of uphill and downhill running into your plan. Don't forget to callous those quads.

➤ Everybody talks about the five major hills on the course. They have names—you know any hill that's named has to be trouble. Cowies, Fields, Bothas, Inchanga, and Polly Shortts are the main culprits, but they aren't the only hills. They're just the only ones with names.

➤ The temperature fluctuation can be drastic over 56 miles. Just because it's hot or cold at the start doesn't mean you won't encounter a big temperature swing in either direction. Consider layering some long sleeves or a light jacket that's easy to shed or carry over your singlet or T-shirt.

➤ Don't forget the metric system. Once again, everything is measured in kilometers, so brush up before you go. Comrades is especially fun because the distance markers go in reverse, so the first one you see lets you know you have 88K to go. It's like the final countdown or something.

➤ While there are aid stations at nearly every mile, remember that you're racing internationally and they don't offer the same kind of refreshments, such as gels, that you can easily find at other races. Bring the fuel you practiced with during training so that you don't end up getting GI distress from something new or different.

➤ You're going to need to do some walking, so don't be afraid to start putting in walking intervals early. Power-walking up the hills is sometimes more efficient than forcing a jog, and it conserves your energy. Alternatively, don't get too excited on any of the early downhill portions. You can do some damage to your legs you'll regret later if you take those too fast.

➤ Take it all in. Truly, this is a major national event, as you'll understand when you get there. Every person in the country is paying attention to the race you're running, so relish it—that rarely (or possibly never) happens in the United States. Engage with the people around you. For most of us, this is a once-in-a-lifetime experience, so enjoy the culture and history behind it. It's remarkable to bear witness.

TRAINING FOR AND RACING ULTRAMARATHONS

Because ultramarathons are considered any distance longer than 26.2 miles, there's a lot of variability in how to prepare for them. The types of races are wide-ranging as well. They can be on roads or trails, flat or hilly, at high altitudes or sea level. They can go straight up mountains or across a desert. Pick your poison—you have many different kinds to choose from.

I recommend that first-time ultrarunners begin by targeting a 50K. It's not too much farther than a marathon but gives you a taste of what's to come if you progress to longer distances. You can use this distance as a stepping-stone to gauge how to alter your training for other races, as well as how to adjust your fueling and nutrition plans, which are critical components of your success.

The truth is, training for a 50K and even a 50 miler is not much different than training for a marathon. You just need an adequate base of mileage underneath you. I recommend that you've finished at least one marathon first and you trained properly for it. If you are consistently comfortable running five times a week and up to 40 miles per week, you are ready to tackle the longer distances.

A Few Tips

➤ **FIGURE OUT YOUR RACING PRIORITIES FIRST.** What time of year do you want to race? Will it be hot or cold? What kind of terrain do you want to cover? Will you need to travel or can you stay at home? Research all your options based on your preferences.

➤ **FIND A COMFORTABLE HYDRATION DEVICE.** Now you really don't have a choice—you have to carry your own nutrition and fluids, which is something you should practice during your long runs. The options abound, of course. There are handheld bottles, there are belts, and then there are backpacks. You have to try a few different options to figure out what meets your needs and can accommodate all your stuff. Go to your local running shop and touch, feel, and try on everything you can.

➤ **EXPERIMENT WITH FOOD.** Some people like "real" food during the longer distances, like sandwiches, fruit, chips, and pretzels. Others like to stick to gels or chews that are typically used in marathons. It's all an individual decision, but knowing that you could be out there for 8 hours (or 2 days, depending on the distance), you can see why you will need to nail down a strategy. You simply can't finish an ultra-distance event without an obscene number of calories consumed along the way.

➤ **TEST YOUR GEAR.** Because ultras can take so many hours to complete, you will also run into all kinds of different weather conditions. Make sure you have tried all the apparel you may need to wear at various times during a race. You will also probably need a few more items, like a trustworthy headlamp for the dark hours and additional shoes and socks for your crew to have ready or to put in a drop bag that's waiting at a certain point on the course.

➤ **BLOCK OUT TRAINING WEEKENDS.** Although you already will have a good sense of the time commitment involved in training after you've done a couple of marathons, the ultra distances can require a bit more on many weekends. Instead of tackling 30 miles in one shot, for instance, it's advisable to set up a few back-to-back long runs of 18 miles on Saturday and 12 miles on Sunday, for example. For most people, these are weekends lost to training, eating, and sleeping. So plan ahead and ask forgiveness from your loved ones.

➤ **TRAIN ON THE RIGHT TERRAIN.** If you're racing on single-track trails, then plan your long runs on single-track trails. If you have signed up for 50 miles of asphalt, train on the roads. If you know the course scales a mountain, have access to a similar ascent for your preparation. Your body needs to know what's coming, so make sure you're getting in a lot of miles on the kind of surface and topography you're going to encounter on race day.

➤ **ADJUST YOUR PACE EXPECTATIONS.** Ultrarunning isn't about splits or what your watch is telling you. If you're coming from a performance perspective in road racing, this can be hard to comprehend. Ultrarunning is based on your perceived effort, and success is nearly never measured in pace per mile, unless you're an elite athlete. Even then, it's a game of intelligence and spreading your effort out to maximize your strengths on the parts of the course that cater to your best skills.

➤ **BE CONSERVATIVE.** If you're new to ultrarunning, it's better to keep your training volume on the lower side instead of increasing it too drastically, which often leads to injury. On long runs, don't worry about how much distance you're covering but instead go by how many hours you're running. It's all about learning to be on your feet for extended periods of time.

➤ **REMAIN CONSERVATIVE ON RACE DAY.** Just like the marathon, the biggest mistake you can make is within the first miles of an ultra. If you feel comfortable, that's a good start, but consider slowing down even more. This is the true meaning of being in it for the "long haul." In a race of 50K, 50 miles, or 100 miles, you want to give yourself every shot possible to cover the distance. Aside from fueling, beginning at a slow pace is one of the best ways to finish successfully.

➤ **KNOW YOUR EXIT STRATEGY.** You thought anything could happen during a marathon? Anything *really* can happen in an ultra. Some days are flawless. Many are not. You'll want to think ahead of time about what situation might warrant your dropping out, then hope you never have to employ the plan. After all the training you put in, usually the only reason to DNF is if you're injured or ill. You're going to feel crushing fatigue, dark moments, and full-body soreness. None of these are reasons to drop out, though. Remind yourself that it's uncomfortable and then get comfortable with that idea.

➤ **RESPECT THE ELEMENTS AND THE LAND.** Unlike the big-city races, you'll be largely on your own out in the wilderness during many ultramarathons. The weather can turn quickly, so be prepared at all times for whatever conditions the region can receive.

Honing Your Hiking Skills

Many ultramarathons occur on mountainous terrain. Even if you register for something flatter, you're still going a long way. You're going to take walking breaks. You should be prepared and plan them ahead of time. Hiking uphill or across technical sections of trail can be more efficient than continuing a slog—plus that slog is probably using up too much of your energy anyway.

Practice hiking during your training so you are using the technique efficiently.

➤ **Plan your walk intervals.** Go into your race with an idea of how you'll use walking or hiking. Some runners know that they're actually quicker hiking uphill than they are running those portions of a race. Or maybe it's a long enough race that you'll simply plan to walk at preset intervals to keep fatigue at bay.

➤ **Practice hiking.** The first time you're trying to run up a hill in the middle of a 50 miler and you get passed by a competitor who's hiking, it will quickly sway your preconceived notions about running at all costs. But you can be sure that the speedy hiker has practiced the technique. It shouldn't really

Also, remember that out in the forest you don't have armies of volunteers cleaning up after you, so don't litter. Pack out whatever you're packing in. Know all the wilderness etiquette that pertains to the setting you're racing in, as well as any wildlife you may encounter (and how to deal with it). Race Web sites are great resources for all this information. Read up and go to the prerace briefing to learn more.

be viewed as a "break" but rather a different method of continuous forward motion. You're saving yourself from some of the muscle fatigue of running, but you still want to maintain your effort level.

➤ **Check your ego.** If the first incline comes at mile three of the race, remember that you will likely thank yourself for hiking it when you're at mile 28 and exhausted. It doesn't matter if you're only 3 miles in or if you're 3 miles from the finish line—hiking will help you get there safely, efficiently, and possibly a little more happily.

➤ **Forget your pace.** Nobody needs to pay attention to any kind of pace-per-mile when they're out on the trails, which is liberating. Again, it's all about effort (it's hard to reinforce this concept enough). Find the most sustainable effort and keep it there for the duration. It doesn't matter what kind of numbers your watch is displaying—the feedback you should be paying attention to is coming from your body, like your breathing, heart rate, and general level of perceived effort.

GATHERING YOUR CREW

In many races, it is advantageous to have a crew, depending on how the course is set up or what the rules of the race are. A crew is a trusty group of friends or family who will meet you at predesignated aid stations to lend support, tough love, your dry shoes, fuel, and nutrition.

I personally like to be self-sufficient. The only time I ever had a crew was during Badwater, but I can see the benefit of having loved ones out on the course to help you achieve your goals. Should you decide to have a crew (or be required to in order to compete), here are a few suggestions regarding whom to pick and how they can best help your efforts.

➤ **CHEMISTRY MATTERS.** Pick people who have a temperament that is even-keeled. The last thing you want is for your support team to lose its marbles if something goes awry. You need rational thinkers working on your behalf when your cognitive abilities begin to falter, which they will at some point during the race. And you want to make sure they are people who get along. This is not the time for drama. Make sure your team works well together or at least can pretend to when you roll into the mile-50 aid station and can't think straight.

➤ **TELL THEM WHAT YOU NEED.** Before race day, have a crew meeting. Show them how you want things set up at the aid stations, give them pointers on what kind of encouragement works for you (tough love? unbridled enthusiasm? quiet words of positivity?), and talk about the tough stuff, like how you'd like them to handle a scenario in which you think you might want to drop out of the race. Tell them under what circumstances that is acceptable to you and under what circumstances they should boot you back on the trail (with love, of course).

➤ **PRINT OUT ALL DIRECTIONS, INSTRUCTIONS, AND RULES.** Many ultras take place in the middle of nowhere. Crews should not rely on GPS or cell phone coverage. Make sure they have hard copies of maps, directions, and important lists of items you will need at each station where you'll see them, and go over all the rules with them. For example, many races only allow the runner to be crewed within a certain distance of the aid station. Some aid stations are not opened for crewing. Sometimes races have strict parking guidelines crews have to follow. You never want to be disqualified from a race because your crew messed up, so go over all these important details before the big day.

➤ **SHOW AND TELL (ABOUT YOUR GEAR).** There's nothing worse than charging into an aid station and handing over your hydration pack to a crew member who has no idea how to fill a bladder. Make sure you go over all your gear, make lists of what you'll need at which aid station, and allow everybody to try it out before race day so they don't flub it when it counts.

➤ **REMIND THEM TO TAKE CARE OF THEMSELVES.** These kind-hearted people are going to be hyper-focused on you and your needs for many hours. The only way they can do that well is if they're taking care of themselves, remembering to eat and hydrate and, in some cases, take naps. Impress upon them the importance of doing what they need to remain happy and enthusiastic. Encourage them to preplan meals and times of the day they will have a window to eat. It's to everybody's benefit that they remain upbeat and well fed.

Sample Ultramarathon Training Plan

(Geared toward a 50-mile race for a new ultrarunner who has experience running marathons. Assumes base of running 40 miles per week and experience running tempos, fartleks, and hill workouts. You should have worked up to a minimum of a 16-mile run before starting this plan.)

	MONDAY	TUESDAY	WEDNESDAY
Week 1	5 miles easy	6 miles easy	Rest day
Week 2	5 miles easy	6 miles easy	Rest day
Week 3	Rest day	5 miles easy	7 miles on hilly terrain
Week 4	Rest day	7 miles on a hilly route	8 miles easy
Week 5	Rest day	7 miles on a hilly route	8 miles easy

THURSDAY	FRIDAY	SATURDAY	SUNDAY
6 miles fartlek: 2-mile warmup 10 x 2 minutes on/90 seconds off 1-mile warmdown	Rest day	3 hours easy	60 minutes easy
6 miles pace workout: 2 miles easy 2 miles at marathon pace 2 miles easy	Rest day	3 hours easy	60 minutes easy
Rest day	8 miles pace workout: 2 miles easy 3 miles at marathon pace 3 miles easy	3 hours easy	75 minutes easy
8 miles pace workout: 2 miles easy 4 miles at marathon pace 2 miles easy	Rest day	3.5 hours easy	75 minutes easy
9 miles speed workout: 2 miles easy 5 miles at marathon pace 2 miles easy	Rest day	3.5 hours easy	75 minutes easy

(continued)

Sample Ultramarathon Training Plan *(cont.)*

	MONDAY	TUESDAY	WEDNESDAY
Week 6	6 miles easy	Rest day	7 miles w/10 x 2-minute hill repeats included in the middle miles
Week 7	Rest day	6 miles easy	8 miles on a hilly route
Week 8	Rest day	9 miles with 10 x 2-minute hill repeats in the middle miles	7 miles easy
Week 9	6 miles easy	Rest day	7 miles easy
Week 10	4 miles easy	Rest day	9 miles on a hilly route

THURSDAY	FRIDAY	SATURDAY	SUNDAY
6 miles easy	8 miles pace workouts: 2 miles easy 4 miles at half-marathon pace 2 miles easy	90 minutes easy	2 hours easy
7 miles easy	9 miles with marathon pace: 2 miles easy 6 miles at marathon pace 1 mile easy	3.5 hours easy	90 minutes easy
6 miles easy	8 miles with pace work: 1 mile easy 6 miles at marathon pace 1 mile easy	4 hours easy	1:45 easy
10 miles w/pace work: 2 miles easy 7 miles at marathon pace 1 mile easy	7 miles easy	2 hours easy	2.5 hours easy
8 miles easy	10 miles with pace work: 1 mile easy 8 miles at marathon pace 1 mile easy	4 hours easy	2 hours easy

(continued)

Sample Ultramarathon Training Plan *(cont.)*

	MONDAY	TUESDAY	WEDNESDAY	
Week 11	Rest day	7 miles easy	8 miles on a hilly route	
Week 12	Rest day	6 miles easy	10 miles on a hilly route	
Week 13	6 miles easy	Rest day	10 miles on a hilly course	
Week 14	Rest day	7 miles easy	12 miles with 12 x 2-minute hill repeats in the middle miles	
Week 15	4 miles easy	Rest day	6 miles on hilly route	
Week 16	6 miles easy	Rest day	4 miles easy	

THURSDAY	FRIDAY	SATURDAY	SUNDAY
7 miles easy	10 miles with pace work: 1 mile easy 8 miles at marathon pace 1 mile easy	4 hours easy	2:15 easy
6 miles easy	10 miles with pace work: 1 mile easy 8 miles at marathon pace 1 mile easy	2.5 hours easy	2 hours easy
8 miles easy	12 miles with pace work: 2 miles easy 9 miles at marathon pace 1 mile easy	4.5 miles easy	2.5 miles easy
6 miles easy	10 miles with pace work: 2 miles easy 7 miles at marathon pace 1 mile easy	2 hours easy	2 hours easy
6 miles easy	8 miles with pace work: 2 miles easy 5 miles at marathon pace 1 mile easy	60 minutes easy	60 minutes easy
Rest day	3 miles easy	Race day	Celebration day

Chapter 8

Training for and Racing Unconventional Events

How to choose unique experiences and why you should add some spice to the calendar

Racing has come a long way since that bare-bones 10K I did in Moore Township. I doubt there was more than one aid station on that course or much water to be found—everybody was so hard core back in the day, or perhaps a little uneducated on how hydration really worked for better performance. Now you can find races that

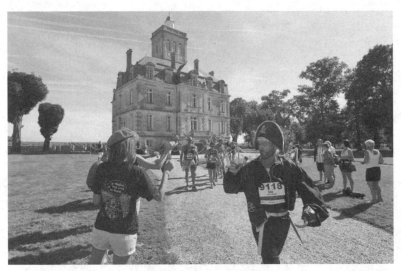
At Le Marathon du Médoc, costumes and wine abound.

offer doughnuts, wine, hot chocolate—whatever your heart desires. You can also find events in exotic locations on the far reaches of the planet, in some of the most challenging geographic landscapes. Running can indeed take us just about anywhere—and I have a bunch of medals and bibs to prove it.

One such race is Le Marathon du Médoc. I've seen a few other events try to imitate it, but you really can't duplicate 21 châteaus through 26.2 miles of French wine country, with 21 wine stops along the way. And that's what this one is, located north of the Bordeaux region. It started in 1984, and the popularity of it grew at the same pace as some of the big-city marathons, though they have to limit it to about 8,500 runners per year. Out of those runners, only a handful show up without a costume, and I can tell you that they must feel desperately out of place. At the starting line when I attended in 2011 they had actors from Cirque du Soleil hanging from a structure 20 feet up, giving people high fives as they set out on the course.

That year the theme of the race was animals. So I had a penguin costume. It was like a onesie almost, except I didn't wear the feet (for obvious reasons). The only problem was that it went up to 90°F that day and I had on this black, one-piece, furry costume, which provided an extra degree of discomfort. Thom Gilligan, the CEO of Marathon Tours, had a gorilla outfit on, so before we began running I thought, "Well, if Thom can run in that gorilla getup, I can certainly handle this penguin outfit." Unbeknownst to me, Thom didn't plan on running the entire race. Around halfway he took his gorilla head off and said au revoir. He was heading back to the finishing area.

The people who organize all the stations along the way really implore each runner to stop at each of the 21 locations to taste a little red or white wine. Runners have to remember to drink water first and eat plenty of crackers so they don't end up in too much trouble. They only pour you about an ounce at each one, but with the heat of the day while you're covering 26.2 miles on foot in a penguin costume, those ounces can add up quickly if you're not careful. You will not go far without refreshments—there are 21 food stands that offer oysters, ham, steak, cheese, and ice cream. I remember getting ice cream at mile 25. It was so good, I ran back and got more. It's a wonder how anybody makes it the whole way. Certainly, many people are not able to do it sober.

The Médoc organizers stay true to their mission: "If you believe sport is synonymous with health, fun, and conviviality, then this marathon is for you," the Web site says. "Spoilsports, thugs, and record seekers are not invited!"

What I enjoy about events like Médoc is that they offer a reason to take ourselves less seriously and enjoy the act of running without being tied to any performance goals. Instead you step outside the norm, experience a new culture, and laugh a lot with people you otherwise wouldn't have met. How many times do we line up at a race with butterflies in our stomachs, our watches at the ready, with a tunnel vision for the finish line? That's not typically the point of unconventional races—the point is to have some fun or take on a one-of-a-kind challenge.

Unconventional events are less about preparation and more about collecting experiences (and stories for your future book). I have collected quite a few that remain highlights of the past four decades of my life.

RACING PIKES PEAK ASCENT AND MARATHON

When I think back on all the races—all of them!—I've done, I've never been as happy as I was at the finish line of Pikes Peak. It was absolutely my favorite marathon of all time, which says a lot. I loved the brutal course, the vibe of the event, the entire race from start to finish.

If you're unfamiliar with Pikes Peak Ascent and Marathon in August, it begins at 6,300 feet above sea level in Manitou Springs, Colorado, which is about 6 miles west of Colorado Springs. Participants run to the summit of Pikes Peak at 14,115 feet, which is 7,815 feet of climbing, then run back down if competing in the marathon option. The average grade going up is 11 percent—which, of course, is challenging on the ascent, but it's brutal in a completely different way on the descent.

The course is mostly on the Barr Trail in Pike National Forest. It's narrow and can be technical with rocks, roots, gravel, and sharp turns. Those who have not run the race within the past 3 years have to qualify to enter by having completed a marathon or longer-distance race in 6 hours or less.

When I ran the marathon in 1991, I did really well going up. I think I was around 25th place at halfway and feeling good. I was looking forward to going downhill because that's what I was good at. What I didn't anticipate was taking a hard fall. I really ripped myself

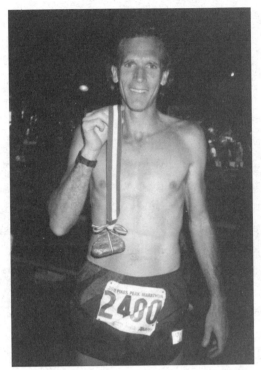

There was joy as well as pain at the Pikes Peak finish line in 1991.

up. The course is tricky because it's a narrow trail and, of course, there are still runners making their way up while you're bombing down. The rules state that the runners coming down have the right of way; however, you never want to take somebody out by accident while you're flying toward the finish. All I remember is stepping on a rock, the rock moving, and the next thing I knew I was down for the count. I got back up, despite being covered in scrapes and impending bruises, and started running again. Then I fell a second time and whacked my hip. I couldn't get my stride back after that.

I just thought I was clumsy and uncoordinated, but when I got to the medical tent and saw how many other runners were in there bleeding, it made me feel better. The medical personnel have these soft-bristle brushes that look like giant toothbrushes to get the stones out of your wounds. The person who was cleaning me up warned me that it was going to hurt, and I said, "I don't feel anything. I'm so high from finishing this race, you could use a wire brush and I wouldn't move." I had gravel in my elbow, shoulder, knee, and ankle. Talk about blood, sweat, and tears—that's Pikes Peak. It lives up to it.

The other part I love about Pikes Peak is staying in Manitou Springs. It's a quaint mountain town where everybody is running or connected to the race. Everywhere you go—every restaurant, coffee shop, ice cream parlor—is filled with runners. There's such a great camaraderie among the people participating and volunteering, you can't help but enjoy it.

I'm a lot slower these days and I start in the second wave for the ascent, which is an option to race the 13.1-mile climb. I did it in 2013 and 2014. At the 5-mile mark of the race, you can hear the announcer at the top calling out the winners crossing the finish line. The sound reverberates off the mountain and you think, "Wow, I'm not going to be there for another 3 hours and these people are already finished." But no matter how long it takes you, few things in life feel more rewarding than climbing up a mountain.

Racing Tips for Pikes Peak

➤ If you're running the ascent race, you can train (mileage-wise) like you would for a regular marathon. You can plan that it will take you about the same amount of time it takes to complete a marathon to finish this race up Pikes Peak. Don't forget to include plenty of climbing in your training plan, of course.

➤ It's critical to begin this race as conservatively as you possibly can. I can't emphasize it enough. Stay well within yourself and do a welfare check every 10 minutes or so. How's your breathing? How's your heart rate? Are you hydrating? Is it time to take a gel? I suggest keeping yourself at as comfortable a pace as you can for as long as you can.

➤ Everybody hikes, unless you're an elite athlete. Even those who are at the front of the pack are going to slow considerably as the terrain gets steeper and the altitude gets higher. Remember that you're trying to conserve energy. At a certain point, hiking is actually faster and more efficient than trying to run.

➤ Be patient. You're on a narrow trail for most of the way and at some point you may want to pass somebody. Wait until the trail widens again if you want to make your move. Otherwise you'll expend a lot of effort to get around people.

➤ The weather will be unpredictable. Prepare for the worst and hope for the best. Some years there is not a cloud in the sky. Other years you'll run into snow squalls as you near the top. Mountain weather can change on a dime and be unforgiving. It's best to carry a waterproof layer with you. The temperature swings from bottom to top can be as much as 50°F.

➤ Keep moving forward. As you climb farther up the mountain, you'll see more of your fellow runners peeling off the trail and taking a seat on a rock. I understand the desire for a break, but I recommend that you keep moving forward. When you sit down, it will be that much harder to get back up. Slow yourself down, walk if it helps, but keep putting one foot in front of the other. Forward march!

➤ Pack warm clothes for the finish line. Again, the temperature above the tree line will be chillier than it was below, and you may be waiting (if you're doing the ascent) for the shuttle bus for a little while before heading back to Manitou Springs.

Running High-Altitude Races

The question I get most often when I talk about Pikes Peak and other races that take place at high altitude is how to prepare for it when you live at sea level?

Why is it so difficult to run at 5,000 feet or more above sea level? Because there is a lower concentration of oxygen, which means your heart and lungs are working a lot harder to get it to your muscles.

You can expect to run anywhere from 20 seconds to a minute slower per mile at high altitude than you do at sea level, and much slower still if you're hitting 10,000 feet or more. If you throw in a lot of hills, you'll go even slower. And that's okay. Guess what? Even people who live at altitude are going slower than they normally would.

The short answer is that you can't prepare if you're only going to be visiting a high-altitude location for a few days. But you can employ a few strategies to cope.

1. **Plan your arrival.** Physiologists say you can acclimate a bit in time for race day if you give yourself about 2 weeks at altitude before the event. With work and other commitments, that's not always feasible. So if it's not, the experts recommend arriving as close to the start time as possible. If you can arrive the previous night and race before you've been there for 24 hours, you can trick your body. Less than 24 hours, it hasn't started processing where you are yet, so you won't feel the fatigue or altitude sickness that some people suffer from after 24 hours.

2. **Hydrate.** The mountains are dry, and you're not always aware of how much you're

RACING IN ANTARCTICA: OR WHEN BART MET SOME ANGRY BIRDS

Traveling to Antarctica to race is about as unconventional as you can get. But because I was granted the opportunity to do just that, I perspiring because it evaporates so fast. Hydration is the key to keeping mountain sickness away, as well as the dehydration headaches some people suffer in the first few days up high. Make sure you're constantly sipping water and sports drinks on your way to the destination and the time leading up to the race.

3. **Get on mountain time.** Not the time zone. I'm talking about lowering your intensity and leaving your watch at home. You have to adjust your expectations and go by effort instead of time. Slow it down and be one with the mountain. I always just try to pay attention to my breathing and heart rate. If you're used to running 7-minute miles on the road at home and you see you're hiking 20-minute miles at 8,000 feet, it can mess with your head. It's best not to know, so you can leave the timing devices at home.

4. **Don't be intimidated.** When people tell me that they'll never consider a race that takes place at high altitude, I am sad for them. You miss a lot of amazing opportunities if you just automatically rule out these experiences. Just do the best you can in your training with what you have. If you're in Florida and targeting Pikes Peak, hop on that treadmill and crank the incline. You can only do so much. Just redefine your expectations and enjoy the views. I promise that you will not regret the decision. Few things are more beautiful than the view from the top of a mountain you just climbed on your own two feet.

can say I've run on all seven continents, which is an accomplishment I'm proud of, and I'm honored to have been given the chance.

The Antarctica Marathon begins with surviving the journey to get there, and I made mine in 1999 with about 170 other runners.

First we met in Buenos Aires, Argentina, to fly to Ushuaia, the capital of the province Tierra del Fuego. It's the world's southernmost city, and it also feels like the end of the earth. From there we boarded a no-frills freight ship, where most of us spent the next 3 days suffering from seasickness as the ship made its way through the Beagle Channel, across the Drake Passage, past the Shetland Islands, and along the Antarctic Peninsula.

The ocean was rough, so getting to our destination took a lot out of almost everybody on board. I decided, in between bouts of illness, to try to run on the deck as we were making our way through the Drake Passage. While I was running around a tiny loop in an attempt to get some fresh air, the ship encountered a 20-foot ocean

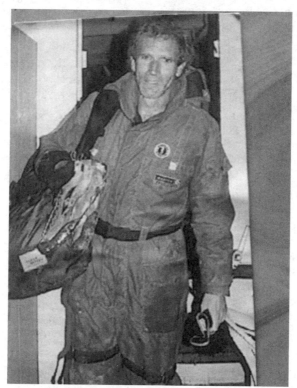

All geared up and disembarking the Zodiac, *Bart prepares to run the Antarctica Marathon.*

swell. I was caught in midair and then slammed back down to the deck as cold ocean water sloshed all around me. That was the end of my running while we were at sea.

When we finally made it to King George Island, we had 2 days to recover from the voyage. I had been recruited to mark the course for the race, so Thom Gilligan, Bill Serues, and I boarded a *Zodiac* (an inflatable boat) carrying a GPS, about 1,000 red flags, some beer, and couple of bottles of vodka. We used four-wheelers to navigate the tundra and to deliver the beer and vodka to Russian scientists at the Bellingshausen Station, where they studied weather and wildlife during the summer months. Most of the people in Antarctica are there to do some sort of research on the bases that are scattered about the area.

As we lined the course with the red flags—which would be the only way the runners would know where to go because there was no existing trail—I had my first encounter with the skuas, predatory birds that nest in that area. I was drilling flags into the tundra when one of the birds came down and whacked me on the head. Then another one. Ouch! Then they started multiplying and coming at me as I covered my head with my arms. To this day, I would rather stand down a bear than deal with one of those birds. They were so aggressive in protecting their nests.

When race day came, it was about 20°F and clear. I ran the half marathon. It was my job before the race to set up the Gatorade and nutrition that the runners supplied for themselves. When we got to mile four, I saw that the food and drinks had been ravaged by those skuas. They had punctured aluminum cans of cola and ripped open PowerBar wrappers, strewing everything all over the place. Our self-serve aid station had been self-served by some angry birds. There was nothing we could do about it at that point—you make do with whatever you have when you're running on Antarctica. Those birds had foiled me again. Luckily, they stayed away from most of the runners during the race. The only ones in danger of attack were the fastest and the slowest—it seemed like the skuas shied away from larger packs, but those running by themselves came under fire.

The race is tough. It offers a little bit of everything at that time of year—we were there in February. There's glacier, as you'd expect, but there's also a decent amount of mud, and some snow. The vastness is the beauty of this place, as well as the wildlife. We saw whales, leopard seals, and penguins—you see an amazing number of penguins on this part of the earth.

So few people ever get to go to this corner of the planet, you really have to take the time to appreciate being there. Nobody goes to set any marathon records, and there's really not much you can do to prepare for a race like this anyway. The weather was akin to a winter day in Chicago, so it wasn't as terrible as many would imagine. One person ran in shorts (there's *always* that person), but the rest of us dressed in layers, including tights, hats, jackets, and gloves. You have to be prepared for a spontaneous whiteout, though we lucked out with the weather that year. The most challenging sections were the fields of deep, sticky mud—the kind that could suck the shoes right off your feet.

Racing Tips for Antarctica

➤ The common theme in any of these unconventional races is to go for the experience and leave the watch at home. That holds true here. The trip is all about bonding with the other runners along the way, seeing a part of the world that few others do, and embracing the fact that your ability to run brought you here. Run the half marathon or the full, but do it for the sheer joy of running somewhere so special.

➤ Since the time that we made the trip, the organization has implemented many new rules to minimize any impact the runners or the event have on the ecosystem. You'll be briefed on all of it before you go, but no nuts or seeds are allowed and littering is, of course, definitely prohibited, for starters.

➤ The other runners also serve as your cheerleaders. The course, though modified several times over the years, is six 4.3-mile loops, which may sound terrible to some people, but you get to go past your aid stations frequently. And because there aren't a lot of people living there to spectate, the runners are the people you get encouragement from. You see them a lot on a short loop.

➤ Antarctica is not flat. The loop contains some decent hills, so be prepared for those. If the temperatures have been warm, the mud is the hardest terrain you'll encounter. It can be thick and difficult to get through at some points.

➤ Everybody takes a *Zodiac* to and from the race. You'll be given a wetsuit and waterproof boots for the voyage to keep you protected from the cold ocean spray.

➤ The event trip sells out years in advance, so if you want to do it, plan ahead and get your name on the list.

RACING THE IRONMAN TRIATHLON

A confession: My life hasn't been entirely spent just running. I've also done my fair share of swimming and biking. In fact, at one point I got proficient enough to string all three disciplines together to race Ironman Canada. And when I did that, I qualified for the 2000 world championships in Kona, Hawaii.

The truth is, I've always been a huge proponent of cross-training, but training for triathlons became more than that for me. I've completed six Ironman distance races (2.4-mile swim, 112-mile bike, 26.2-mile run), including Lake Placid, New York; Wisconsin; Canada; and Kona.

I will admit that when I was focused on preparing for these races, it was tough to stay on track because I traveled so much for work. When you're training just for running events, you only need to pack some shorts and shoes. When you need to bike and swim, it requires a whole different level of planning and forethought while you're out of town. I tried to swim twice a week, I commuted to and from work on my bike when I was home, and then, of course, continued on with my usual running routine. Somehow it all came together for me.

You learn pretty quickly that you spend the most time during the race on the bike. Luckily, I was already skilled at long-distance cycling. And being a runner by trade meant that I had a lot of good muscle memory in my legs. The weakest discipline for me was the swim. I really never invested the necessary time in getting much better at it—though, like many triathletes, I got away with it because it's the shortest part of the race.

Ironman Canada, which now takes place in Whistler, British Columbia, was my favorite because the bike course was challenging and the feel of the town was similar to Manitou Springs at Pikes Peak. At that time it was based in Penticton, and everybody there was either competing or connected to the race. It felt enthusiastic and supportive, which is a nice vibe when you're embarking on such a daunting goal. To me, Canada was even better than Kona, which is the race everybody associates with Ironman, of course.

At the Canada race, my most vivid memory was on the bike, climbing up Richter Pass, a mountain pass that links the Similkameen Valley with the South Okanagan. It started sleeting, and we were getting pelted with hail at the top. While most people probably wouldn't enjoy it, I thought it was awesome. It didn't seem to make the road too slick, which was a good thing; it just made the entire experience more interesting. I loved it.

Kona, however, has the mystique and the prestige—it's a big deal to qualify to race there.

Kona reminds me a lot of the Boston Marathon, though it has a young history in comparison. It's a gathering of the best triathletes in the world. I was struggling with my Lyme disease at the time, but I was convinced it would be my only opportunity to race there, so I decided to give it a go. I wanted to give it my best shot no matter how I was feeling, mostly because you never know if you're going to get to do it again.

I survived the swim, which is as treacherous as everybody makes it out to be. You get beat up and run over by all those fellow competitors. It's rough. It's like swimming inside a washing machine. I was glad to finish it and get on my bike—my only goal for those 112 miles was just to keep it rolling without incident. The more relaxed you can stay on the bike ride, the better off you'll be. It's also a critical time to pay attention to your fueling and hydration plan.

What I didn't expect was that the run would be so difficult. It was harder than I thought it would be. It wasn't so much the heat, which is always a factor in Hawaii; I just wasn't feeling it that day. But I had made a pact with myself that I had to do this race before I was unable to participate in this level of competition anymore. So I tried to take it in and appreciate it for what it is. You can't help but think about all those early images of the sport playing out right on the ground you're racing, like the 1980s, when Dave Scott just dominated the podium each year and became a legend.

So why would a runner want to take time away from concentrated training? I get this question often from the diehards out there. Runners notoriously hate cross-training. But I like going fast on a bike and the ability to mix things up. Adding in cycling and swimming can also keep you in the running game longer. They add strength and cardiovascular fitness in a nonimpactful way, which can only make you better for longer and probably less injury-prone. Granted, while you're training for something as long and grueling as Ironman, your running speed will suffer and deteriorate. It doesn't last forever. Putting in a lot of cycling miles will slow you down as a runner, but when you get back to full-focused running, it comes back quickly, plus you've built a lot of strength in other ways that can only improve your athleticism.

And who knows? You might find out you're good at triathlon. I used to win a lot of them, which motivated me to do more. And taking a hiatus from running will often make us hungrier when we come back to it.

Triathlon Tips for Runners

➤ For those who are performance-minded, you have to change your attitude. You might be a great runner, but you might not be the greatest runner after you get off your bike. Don't let it defeat you—it's just another way to challenge yourself.

➤ Don't start with the Ironman. Just like I advise new runners to start with a 5K, it's best for new triathletes to begin with sprint and Olympic distance triathlons, which are much shorter but still give you a sense of the difficulty of the sport. And perhaps that will be enough for you. Either you'll catch the fever and want to progress to a half Ironman and Ironman or you'll call it good. It's best to figure that out gradually.

➤ Forget mileage. Triathletes don't measure their training in miles, they measure it in hours. And when you begin, you'll want to focus more of the hours on the bike and swim—train your weaknesses, not your strengths. We always gravitate to what we're good at, but that doesn't help us get better at the other disciplines.

➤ If you're really bad at swimming, take a lesson. Almost every community has a YMCA or similar recreation center where skilled swim coaches are available to help with a private lesson or two. Take advantage because form is what will make your swimming performance improve—you actually can't get any faster without a pretty stroke. If you've already got enough technique to stay afloat and move forward, consider joining a masters swim team, which is led by a coach. Swimming is much easier when you don't have to think about your workout yourself. Without prior competitive swimming experience, it's difficult to know how to frame a productive workout. Note that "masters" in swimming does not mean the same age group that it does in running—anybody older than 18 can join a masters swimming group.

➤ You could spend a fortune on a bike and all the other triathlon gear. Don't do that until you are certain you're going to pursue this newfound passion with enthusiasm over a few years. If you already have a bike, no matter how lame it is, just use it for a while and ignore anybody who dares to poke fun at your steed. If you become interested in doing more, then it becomes more necessary to research all the road and tri-bike options. The most important aspect is that your bike fits you. Many people have a professional measure all the dimensions and make the necessary adjustments. You want that bike to feel comfortable—if it doesn't, you won't want to ride, and you'll also risk injury.

➤ Slow down your runs. This might be a challenge for those who have spent years doing everything in their power to get faster on foot. But now you have a lot more on your plate, so you have to slow down your training to conserve your energy. Also, note that when you're racing this portion of a triathlon, you probably just won't have the leg speed you're used to. After all, you've already had quite a workout before it even starts.

➤ Decrease your running mileage. Adding two swims and many hours of biking to your routine will naturally cut down on your running. Don't panic. You still get to run, just not as far or maybe as often.

➤ Fuel up. Unless you've mastered the ultramarathon, you have no idea how much more you need to take in when you are racing triathlons. But just like increasing racing distance in running,

Basic Triathlon Gear Requirements

Many runners avoid trying triathlons because the gear can seem overwhelming. You don't need to invest in everything right away, and you certainly do not need the best of any of it, either. Here are the basics that I recommend.

Swim

1. **Wetsuit.** Many triathlon swims take place in open water. If the temperature is cool, you'll want a wetsuit. Not only will it keep you warm, it will also add to your buoyancy. Practice in it to be sure it fits correctly—it can feel restrictive, and if you're nervous, it might seem suffocating if it isn't the proper size. Some local shops will rent wetsuits, which could be a better option if you don't want to purchase one.

2. **Goggles.** Make sure you've tried out your goggles in training. You don't want to experience leaks during your race.

Bike

1. **Bike.** Any kind that gets you from point A to point B is fine. If you end up falling in love with bicycling, then you'll go on a hunt for one in much the same manner you shop for a car. And you can spend just as much money on it if you want to. Just make sure whatever you're using fits your body.

experimenting with all the fueling options in triathlon takes time. It's convenient to do most of the intake on the bike. You're doing this portion the longest, so it's necessary to keep the glycogen stores topped off. And you definitely don't want to bonk when you hit the run.

➤ Learn how to negotiate transitions. The time between the swim, bike, and run counts toward your overall results, so many

There is nothing worse than a bad bike fit, and nothing will make you avoid riding more than feeling uncomfortable.

2. **Flat kit.** You have a flat to look forward to—it happens to everybody. Carry a kit that contains everything you need to fix it and learn how to do so before it happens in a race.

3. **Helmet.** Not much more to say other than it needs to fit properly and be comfortable. Protect your brain.

4. **Sunglasses.** They aren't just needed to look cool or take the glare off, though it's important to protect your eyes from the sun. On a bike, they also pro-

tect your baby blues (or hazels or browns) from gravel and bugs that may be kicked up along the way.

5. **Hydration bottles.** You'll want multiple bottle holders attached to your bike. Make sure your hydration devices fit securely in them so they don't bounce out and roll away.

Run

1. **Shoes.** I'm going to assume you know this part.

2. **Sunglasses.** Again, they're good protective wear. I made the mistake of not wearing them most of my life and I'm paying for it now.

triathletes have to practice those, too. During your first few races, they can be awkward. You'll learn how to organize your transition area after a couple of tries. In training, it's fun to practice transitions when you are doing an open-water swim (like at a lake). Get out of the water, strip off your wetsuit, get the socks, shoes, sunglasses, helmet, and gloves on, and ride away.

➤ Always remember in the second transition: Take your bike helmet off before you start the run. You wouldn't believe how many people forget to do this.

Chapter 9

Training for and Racing Relays and Multiple Race Events

How to make a race a team sport and why you should add a few distances to your weekend challenge

Back in the late 1980s, I did the Gasparilla Distance Classic, which is a 15K in Tampa, on a Saturday and then decided to do a 5K in Fort Myers that night. It was long before anybody considered doing more than one race in two days, let alone two in one day, and everybody thought I was a lunatic. I did it because I had *Runner's World* work obligations at both events, so I didn't see why I shouldn't run both races. I understood at the time that it was unusual, but it was also fun.

Little did I realize I was just ahead of my time, although I do recall in the early 1980s that some people did an event with 5 races in 2 days—from 100 meters up to the marathon. But it all became mainstream in 2006 when the Walt Disney World Marathon decided to create Goofy's Race and a Half Challenge. The event director, John Hughes, told me he thought perhaps 200 people might sign up to run the half marathon on Saturday and the marathon on Sunday just to earn the bragging rights and a Goofy medal. He was wrong. The first year, about 3,000 people registered for the challenge and an entirely new racing event was born. Since then, Walt Disney World has added the Dopey Challenge, which includes running the 5K, 10K, half marathon, and marathon over the 4 days of the event.

Why have these multirace events taken off? I believe it's the bling and swag. All the medals and T-shirts runners earn for completing these feats are attractive to more people than I ever realized. Like all new challenges, runners began flocking to them because they were an opportunity to notch novel and unique accomplishments. Now the options seem endless—including right here at the *Runner's World* Half Marathon and Festival, where we offer incentives for completing combinations of the trail run, 5K, 10K, and half marathon throughout the weekend. Runners tell me that when they travel somewhere, they want do it all—and if you attach a clever name to it like Goofy, Dopey, Hat Trick, Five & Dime, or Grand Slam, it just seems to add to the allure. We actually had to educate people about what a Hat Trick is at our *Runner's World* event. Apparently runners don't watch a lot of hockey.

Through the years, relays have increased in popularity as well. One of my favorites happens to be one of the originals—the Hood to

Coast Relay, where 12-person teams run 199 miles, from the Timberline Lodge at Mount Hood, in Oregon, to Seaside. In 1995, *Runner's World* sent a bunch of teams to compete and it ended up providing one of my most memorable racing moments. I was running one of my legs and clicking off 5:10 miles like clockwork, feeling pretty good about myself.

My legs were fresh—one of those runs that felt effortless. Then I saw this shadow moving in on me, closer and closer. I couldn't imagine who might be going faster at that point. Well, it was Alberto Salazar. You know, the guy who won the New York City Marathon three times and the 1982 Boston Marathon? After a hiatus from the sport, Alberto was back into running—he had just won Comrades and on this particular night in Oregon he and his team, named Mambu Baddu (Swahili for "the best is yet to come"), was on the way to winning Hood to Coast and smashing the course record. That group finished in 15:45:55, which meant they averaged 4:51 per mile over 199 miles. That's cruising.

Anyway, Alberto was flying. He zipped right past me like I was

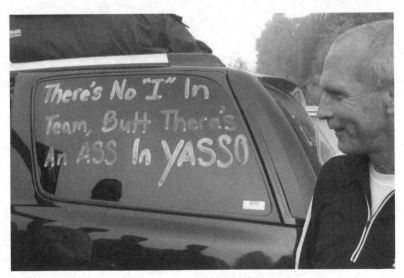

Feeling the team love at the Hood to Coast Relay.

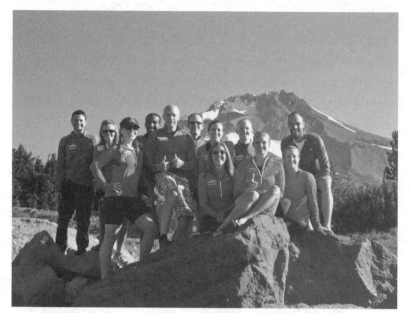

From Hood...

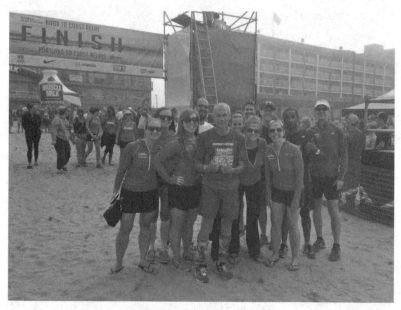

... to Coast, with the Runner's World *team.*

stuck in the mud. To me it was the coolest thing. When was I ever going to be in front of Alberto Salazar in a race again? His team started about 2 hours after ours did. That's one of the attractions of Hood to Coast—you just never know who else is going to be out there. I enjoy the chaos of that event. It's a scavenger hunt, race, and party all at the same time, just rolling down the road to the beach.

The common tie between relays and multirace event weekends is that you have to manage your effort level appropriately across a couple of days and various running distances, usually with some sleep deprivation mixed in. If you start hammering at your first race or relay leg of the weekend, you're probably setting yourself up for a degree of personal disaster. Everybody is different in how they respond to this kind of racing stress, but I can tell you that when you get a bunch of runners together doing something slightly crazy with very little sleep, you will make some memories and have a lot of laughs. And maybe a few tears, too.

One recollection I go back to time and again when I'm thinking about all the varieties of races I've done is during the Ragnar Relay in 2013 from Miami to Key West, Florida, which unfortunately has since been discontinued due to local government permitting issues. After we got out of the urban area and made our way through the Keys, we were running over narrow bridges with nothing blocking the horizon in any direction. The sun was setting on our right as the moon simultaneously rose on our left. It was a breathtaking, unobstructed sight over the water—one of those moments when I especially appreciated the natural beauty that running brings into our lives.

Indeed, some of my best experiences in the sport have been due to these unique racing opportunities. They're obvious ways to infuse fun into a routine. Most of us are guilty of becoming so focused on personal records and performance for long stretches of time, it's easy to start feeling burned out or fatigued and forget that running is supposed to enhance our quality of life. It's refreshing and rejuvenating to keep in touch with the pure enjoyment of the sport. It's also nice to challenge ourselves in new or different ways—and completing 48.6 miles of racing in 4 days through Walt Disney World is one of many ways to do that.

BART'S FAVORITE RELAY: HOW TO TRAIN FOR AND RACE HOOD TO COAST

When Bob Foote started Hood to Coast, which takes place in August, he was actually in need of a new running challenge. He gathered up a bunch of friends to run from Mount Hood to the beach, each taking turns along the way. In 1982, eight teams of 10 runners ran 5-mile legs of the course to complete the first edition of the storied event. Then the word spread, and now it's nearly impossible to gain entry—teams have to enter a lottery to be selected.

These days, teams are comprised of 12 members in two vans and the legs are of varying distances. The starting times at the Timberline Lodge are staggered from 5 a.m. until 3 p.m. so that the route has a steady flow of vans and runners. Getting a team organized can be the hardest part—figuring out which runner is taking which legs is like putting a puzzle together. The course has many sections that may not be the longest mileage, but cover the most difficult terrain. You'll find significant descents early on, which can ruin quads for later. There are sections that are exposed to the sunshine, should that be a factor, and stretches of gravel instead of paved road. The race provides a cheat sheet that evaluates the difficulty level and mileage for each runner, which makes it a bit easier to assign everybody legs that more or less cater to their strengths. This is all part of the fun, of course.

How to Train for Hood to Coast

Depending on the degree of your team's competitive spirit, preparing for a relay race should feel less intense than many other races. But there are a few aspects to incorporate into about 6 weeks of training before race day.

1. **KNOW YOUR RELAY LEGS.** The Hood to Coast course has a bit of everything included in it, so if your duties include some screaming downhill portions, you're going to want to prepare your quads to absorb the shock (see my downhill training tips in Chapter 6). If it's likely you'll be racing at least once during the hottest part of the day, you should incorporate some training in the heat, if possible. Just look at all the information provided about the course, organize your team early, and prepare yourself for your responsibilities.

2. **TRAIN MULTIPLE TIMES A DAY.** About once a week for 6 weeks consider running before work, at lunch, then after work to simulate the condensed rest between runs that you'll have during the race. Your body will begin to adapt to the process. During these days you'll figure out what to eat, how much, and when so that you feel fueled but you don't experience any GI distress. You'll learn to hydrate well between runs and perhaps take some time to foam roll and stretch, too, so that when you're sitting at your desk all day (kind of like sitting in a cramped van all day), you'll be less likely to stiffen up. These once-a-week experiments will teach you everything you will need to do, drink, and eat during the race.

3. **RUN IN THE DARK.** Chances are you'll have at least one leg in the dark. Many people have never run in nondaylight hours. Get a headlamp and practice because it can be an odd feeling—to some people it may feel a bit dizzying at first. It takes some

adaptation to run by the light of a headlamp. You don't want to do that for the first time at a race.

4. **MAKE A PLAN.** Communicate with the team and set expectations appropriately. It's important that everybody be on the same page regarding strategy. Most groups are just out there for the fun and camaraderie. Other teams might be going for Alberto-like speed. Whatever the philosophy is, make sure the whole group is in agreement while preparing for the race. There's nothing worse than showing up at Mount Hood having not prepared adequately to pull your weight on a team going for the podium.

Racing Tips for Hood to Coast

When you make it to Mount Hood, everybody will be fresh. Your van won't smell like dirty runner yet. Energy will abound. Capture that moment. It's the last time you'll see everybody looking so put together.

Hopefully, before you've arrived, you've already divided the group up into two vans. You've come up with a driver schedule (if you haven't appointed two nonrunners to drive), and your bags are ready to go.

Runner No. 1 is off, and the rest of the team is following the agreed-upon plans of action.

➤ **EASY DOES IT.** The first three runners need to take it easy. They'll be running the group down the mountain, and it's steep. There's no reason to push the pace—just let gravity do the work. Resist breaking. Flow down the hills and save yourself for the next leg.

➤ **TAKE CATNAPS.** The urge to stay awake and cheer on your teammates is strong. There will be plenty of time for that, but if

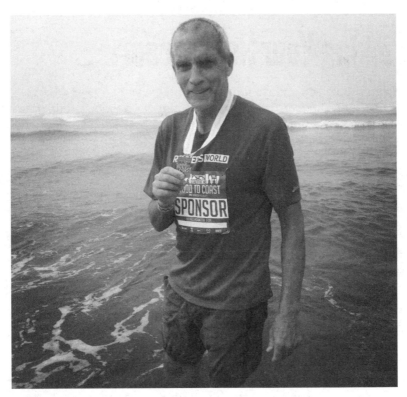

Bart partakes in nature's ice bath on the coast of Oregon.

you feel like you can catch a few z's at any point, do it. Essentially, you'll be awake from Friday morning until Saturday night, so start napping early, even after the beginning legs, if you can.

➤ **EAT, DRINK, EAT, DRINK.** Stuff the van with all the snacks you can—and, of course, try to stick to the kinds of foods you practiced in training. Whenever the opportunity arises, eat something small. Don't be shy with the carbs and have protein options available, too, like peanut butter. Don't let yourself get hungry. As soon as you finish a leg, start rehydrating with sports drinks and water.

➤ **STRETCH AND ROLL.** After you're done running your first and second legs, go for a cooldown jog for a few minutes, then stretch

Picking Your Relay Team

Whom should you choose for your squad? There are many ways to create a team, but it's most critical that everybody agrees what the goals are: fun or competition? Most likely you're in this for the fun.

The most successful relay events that I've taken part in are when I've found myself on a team of people who are about my same ability. If we're all likely going to be running the same pace—or within 15 seconds per mile faster or slower—things tend to go smoothly. We know when to anticipate arrivals, we know roughly where we'll place in the pack, and we know how to assign legs to the group. It's just easier when you're all similar runners.

That doesn't mean a team has to be chosen that way, however. Plenty of groups gather up friends with great chemistry and see where the chips fall. Others don't care if they're all best friends, they just want the fastest possible team they can muster. It all depends on what kind of experience you're after—your team will be the most critical factor in that, of course.

Another thing to note is that you're going to need some alternate members. When race registrations open, everybody is excited to join the fun. As race day nears, however, people will be sick, injured, or have unexpected personal matters that force their cancellation. Have a few people ready to take their place—most likely you're going to need to call them.

and foam roll as much as you can before you stuff your smelly self back into the van. This all jump-starts the recovery process so that you're not starting out in bad shape for your next leg.

➤ **ARRIVE TO EXCHANGE POINTS EARLY.** You don't want to stress anybody out, so don't dawdle getting to the exchange zones. Leave enough time for bathroom stops, a light warmup jog, and a little more stretching and foam rolling, if you have time. Do a gear check to make sure you have everything you need with you. For example, if the sun is going to set during your leg, you'll need a headlamp, extra batteries, and reflective clothing.

➤ **STAY DRY.** Pack enough clothing so that you can change out of sweaty shirts and shorts as soon as you're done with a leg. The last thing you want is to catch a chill or just feel uncomfortable between legs. Besides, the more stench you're wearing, the more stench you're sharing with your teammates.

➤ **KEEP TABS ON EACH OTHER.** Remember this is a team sport. Make sure to ask how everybody is feeling and try to keep your crew upbeat. If the driver looks tired, come up with a way to give him or her a break. Have each other's backs and keep things light—that's when you're most likely to make good memories.

WHAT TO PACK FOR RELAY WEEKEND

When you have 12 team members, two vans, and a lot of snacks and drinks to lug, it's suggested that you pack as lightly as you can. To save redundancies, remember you can share stretching ropes, foam rollers, yoga mats, and other self-massage tools. Come up with a big list of groceries for everybody to share so 12 people don't bring 24 bags of food or 10 cases of sports drinks.

A few other items to put in your bag, besides your running shoes and racing attire:

➤ Three sets of clothes for in between running legs. Consider dividing them into labeled plastic bags so that they're easily accessible and organized.

➤ Hat, sunscreen, and sunglasses

➤ Deodorant, toothbrush, toothpaste, travel-size personal hygiene products as needed

➤ Comfortable shoes for in between legs

- Extra socks and underwear

- A backup pair of running shoes

- Waterproof layers, including a lightweight wind jacket

- Headlamp and extra batteries; taillight

- Chargers for all devices

- Reusable water bottle

- Small pillow and blanket

- Shower wipes

- Hand sanitizer

- Towel

- Antichafing balm

- Reflective safety vest

- Watch

TRAINING FOR AND RACING MULTIDISTANCE EVENTS

Getting ready for something like the Dopey Challenge is a lot like preparing for a relay. You have to get the body adapted to running in a fatigued state, which requires a few weekends of back-to-back training runs.

If you're aiming for a challenge that's higher mileage, like running a 5K, 10K, half marathon, and marathon, you don't need to complete those distances in training, of course. But consider building in peak weeks of running, when you plan to do 3 miles on Thursday, 4 miles on Friday, 6 miles on Saturday, and 16 to 18 miles on Sunday. During the weeks that you implement this kind of consecutive mileage, make sure to take 2 rest days.

During those back-to-back runs, you're trying to simulate how the race weekend will go. You'll learn how to keep your pace slow and conservative in the first two runs, which will allow you to appropriate your energy over the long haul and sustain the even effort throughout. It may take a little bit of trial and error to get it right, but my advice is to run exceedingly slow to be on the safe side.

During those weekends you'll also rehearse your hydration, eating, and sleeping routines. All of these activities have amplified importance when you're competing in a multirace event. You're only going to be as good as your recovery allows you to be, so make sure you're getting plenty of sleep during the nights, naps during the day (if you can), and lots of postrun carbs and protein-rich meals. You'll want to constantly sip on water and sports drinks between efforts, too. During your training, you'll figure out the timing and the ingredients for your most effective recovery methods. And while it's hard not to get distracted by the surroundings of your race, try to stick to the routine as best you can during the event.

The good news is that the courses for the Disney races are all similar and relatively flat. You're not going to need to prepare for tough terrain. Other setups aren't as forgiving. Take the *Runner's World* Half and Festival, for example. If you're partaking in the Grand Slam, which is a 3.8-mile trail race, 5K, 10K, and half marathon for 26.2 miles over 3 days, you're going to deal with a lot of hills on all the courses. The 5K and 10K aren't spaced that far apart on Saturday, so the relaxation time between them is quick. The weekends that you set aside for more intense training should include some hilly terrain so that your legs are ready to power through the undulating streets of Bethlehem, Pennsylvania.

Tips for Racing Weekend

➤ What I find most difficult for the Walt Disney World challenges is the sleep deprivation. The wake-up calls and starting times are all extremely early, so by Sunday, when you're toeing the line for 26.2 miles, you can be pretty exhausted. Try to get into the habit after the first race of taking a nap during the day. The shut-eye will pay off.

➤ Think of the 5K and 10K as glorified shakeout runs for the half marathon and marathon. Whatever distances you're racing—or however many events—you want the first two to be extremely slow. For example, if your marathon pace is 10:00 miles, then run the 5K and 10K at 10:15 per mile pace, then in the half marathon and marathon try for 10:00 pace. That's how I completed the Goofy Challenge, and it worked. If you do it the other way it won't work—most people are unable to start out at goal pace and sustain it through 4 days of racing.

➤ Get into a postrace routine that jump-starts recovery every day. As soon as you cross the finish line, stretch, foam roll, hydrate, and eat. If you feel as though you've just been on an easy run, that's a good sign, but don't let that feeling trick you into believing you don't need to take all the necessary steps to helping your body repair itself.

➤ During the day's race, you should get a head start on the following day's work by taking in fuel. If you take in a gel or other nutrition while you're running, you'll stave off depletion. If you're not exactly craving chews or gels, take them in anyway. It's money in the bank.

➤ Before you go to bed, make sure to stretch and foam roll again. I've learned the hard way if you go to bed achy and stiff, you'll wake up achier and stiffer. Do whatever you can to loosen the legs up before you fall asleep. There's nothing worse than waking up at 3 a.m. for the next race unable to get out of bed without wincing.

➤ Bring two pairs of racing shoes. You never know when one will get wet or damaged.

➤ It's hard to set personal records at any distance for these kinds of challenges, but it's wise to think about goals for each distance. If you're really hoping to run one of them at your fastest pace, then choose which one is most realistic and important to you.

➤ Break the mileage down into easily digestible chunks. Don't think of the Dopey Challenge, for example, as 48.6 miles. Break it down by 5Ks if that helps, or two shakeout runs and a hard training weekend. Whatever way you need to cut it up to make it seem less overwhelming is a good solution.

Chapter 10

Building Longevity for the Long Run

Advice from somebody who knows how to stay in the game for more than four decades

After 40 years, more than 1,200 races (and counting!), and an untold number of miles logged, I often wonder how my body has allowed me to stay upright and moving forward for so long. Many of my health problems may have deterred others from continuing on in the sport—and there have been plenty of moments I thought I was done—but my love for running hasn't let up, so I haven't either. Granted, my tolerance for pain is unusually high, almost to a fault, and nearly to my early demise. But my heart and head have led the way. My legs have merely followed.

Running is a game of balance. If you want to keep doing it for as long as I have, you need to constantly look at the bigger picture. Injuries and illnesses can take you out at the most heartbreaking times, but it's how you cope with them that determines your longevity in the sport. Every obstacle is more like a crossroads—pushing through often makes the challenges insurmountable. The worst examples of stubbornness can be career ending. It's riding a fine line between working hard and overdoing it. It's the smart decisions we make at these junctures that lead to consistency, health, and longevity.

Your running life, like mine, will go through seasons. When I started, I was motivated by competitive goals. I wanted to beat my brother George. Then I wanted to qualify for the Boston Marathon. I wanted to get faster and I wanted to win. I held on tight to my mileage, my workout paces, my racing schedule. Most of my routine revolved around my running performance. It's what got me hooked and kept me engaged for many years, even after Lyme disease made it more difficult.

When I returned from Mount Kilimanjaro, I went through a long course of recovery and antibiotics to try to rebuild the strength that the disease had stolen—it's a scene that's played out three times in my running life. But that time it was significant, sort of a line in the sand. Just 13 weeks later I was on the starting line of the Chicago Marathon to pace the 3-hour group. Getting to that race and helping a bunch of people achieve a goal was my motivation to get back into shape after that horrible episode in Tanzania. And after we crossed the finish line in 2:59:30, I knew I needed to pick another race, but one that was just for me.

So I headed to the Smoky Mountain Marathon in Tennessee. It was a scenic course with terrain that took away all the pressure to chase a specific time. I knew those PR days were over for me. I trained hard, but ran less. I left my watch at home more often than

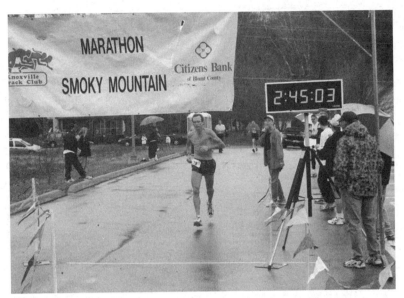

After Bart's health took a hit, he found personal victory in the Smoky Mountains.

not. I took in the surroundings on runs I had done thousands of times, but I had never really seen. Then I drove to Tennessee with the idea of hiking the hilly stretches of the route and running the rest. My only goal was to cover 26.2 miles.

The day of the Smoky Mountain Marathon, with a year of turmoil behind me, I approached the challenge with a degree of patience and calmness that marked a new era in my running career. And perhaps in this I learned a truth: that the tighter you cling to something, the harder it is to hold on to. I had loosened my grip on running, finally, and by mile 20 I was leading the race. Who would have thought? Certainly not me. At age 43 I won my first marathon.

My health has forced me to constantly redefine the role that running plays in my life. Everybody has an evolution and journey of their own, for reasons that are as varied as why we all enter this sport at all. The common denominators I've found in achieving a lifetime of running are an ability to listen to your body and the confidence to step away temporarily—not only when you're forced to because of sickness or injury, but also when you feel the urge to try something new. Some of those breaks for me, like focusing on Ironman or riding my bike across the country, have given me the experiences of a lifetime and the ability to return to running refreshed and rejuvenated. In its absence you can regain a perspective on why you love it and how you want to approach it.

Despite joint pain and a damaged right leg—caused by Lyme, which manifests in a limp even when I'm walking—I still love to line up at many races. Besides changing my mindset, I have also embraced a method that allows me to keep going. Jeff Galloway started his run/walk method of racing years ago and it's helped me tremendously. The key has been to figure out the run/walk ratio that works best for my goals. If I want to break 5 hours in the marathon, I run 3 minutes and walk 1 minute. I tend to run/walk for the first 13.1 miles, and if I'm feeling good, I'll run the entire second half of the marathon. It goes to show that if you're adaptable and keep an open mind, you can keep rolling for many years.

I don't pretend to have some magic formula for running forever—if I did, I'd patent it and make a lot of money. But I have gleaned a bit of wisdom along the way that might help prolong your time and enjoyment in the sport. I thought that Comrades would be my last hurrah, and here I am 7 years later, still finishing marathons. I may not run fast, I may not have the perfect form, but I still love every step.

STRENGTH TRAINING

More runners seem to understand the significance of strength training now than they did many years ago. We've learned that this kind of supplemental work can reduce injury risk, improve running economy, and contribute to good running posture, too. Not only that, but it builds the muscles' ability to sustain a given pace longer—the stronger you are, the less likely it is that you'll start breaking down in the later stages of a race. Resistance training just generally helps our bodies to better absorb the impact of all the pounding we do on the roads, track, and trails. And let's face it—it also burns calories and helps us stay lean.

I've always tried to get to the gym about twice a week. While I'm there, I focus on strength and flexibility. The strength-training part of my routine is fairly simple. I tend to focus on exercises that help build up the stabilizer muscles and tendons—the ones that support the muscles we primarily use for running.

We all have so many choices right now for ways to incorporate strength training. You don't have to merely hit the weight room and do deadlifts by yourself anymore if that doesn't appeal to you. Now you can try CrossFit, yoga, barre, Pilates—whatever floats your boat. I've tried all of them, and my only advice is to find something that you enjoy because if you like what you're doing, you're more likely to stick to it and reap the benefits.

As we age we know that our muscle mass and bone density begin to deteriorate. Running alone won't stave off that process, which is another reason we should all get in the habit of supplemental resistance training no matter what age we are. Research and theories abound about what's best—high reps with low weight or low reps with high weight. My theory, based on no research, is anything is better than nothing. And body-weight exercises are great, too. If you're new to a routine, start conservatively, focus on performing the correct form, and increase the difficulty level as your body adjusts to it.

Experts recommend hundreds of different kinds of strength exercises for runners. I've learned that 30 minutes about twice a week works for me. The only way for a strength routine to be successful and achieve its purpose is if you're consistent about it.

Change it up every month to keep your mind engaged and to make sure you're not plateauing.

The right kind of exercises for runners won't just work one muscle at a time—the exercises that will do the most good will engage multiple groups of muscles at once.

Here are a few of the basic moves to consider when you are putting together a strength routine. There are countless variations of all exercises and many more to explore—make sure you're performing anything you choose correctly and asking for expert assistance at your local gym if you need guidance.

- ➤ Basic planks and side planks
- ➤ Bicycles
- ➤ Superman
- ➤ Russian twists
- ➤ Mountain climbers
- ➤ Bridges
- ➤ Classic pushups
- ➤ Body-weight squats (include single leg)
- ➤ Lunges
- ➤ Burpees
- ➤ Hamstring curls with physio ball
- ➤ Pullups
- ➤ Dips
- ➤ Calf raises
- ➤ Dumbbell squats to press
- ➤ Dumbbell bench press

FLEXIBILITY

I can't think of anything that runners are worse at than touching their toes. We just aren't a flexible people. Most marathoners couldn't jump over the Sunday newspaper on the driveway.

Flexibility in running increases our range of motion, and some forms of stretching indeed keep us injury-free, but we don't have any need to achieve Gumby status. If we get too limber, we lose a bit of our efficiency while running. But if we get too stiff, we can't get out of bed. This is a tricky balancing act.

Gone are the days when we used static stretching on cold muscles before a run. Now the research shows that it's best to use a dynamic warmup that includes flexibility to prime the muscles for the workout ahead. What does that mean? Well, many of the strength exercises that use body weight are also incorporating the right amount of flexibility work, plus they're active instead of passive sit-and-stretch motions. Save the yoga moves for after your run. Beforehand, do some exercises that wake up the muscles that have been sleeping all day at your desk—walking lunges, squats, leg swings, donkey kicks, high knees, and the like will all achieve these goals.

Another popular way to work flexibility using a dynamic routine is learning active isolated stretching (AIS), which you perform with a rope. This can be done whenever you want—before a run, after a run, while you're watching television at night, or right before you go to bed. The basic premise of AIS is that you're isolating the muscle you're stretching by actively contracting their opposite muscles. For example, if you want to stretch your hamstring, you first contract your quad, which will relax your hamstring. You don't hold any stretch more than 2 seconds and you repeat about 10 times. Gradually the range of motion improves and you can quickly move through the routine.

Me? I just start every run at a slow pace, so the first 10 to 12 minutes is what I consider a gradual, easy stretch. Life moves at a frantic pace, so slow down a bit when it comes to running. We runners may not be able to touch our toes, but the good news is that we don't really have to. If you're consistently strength training and implementing a short, dynamic warmup before your runs, you're probably doing enough.

CROSS-TRAINING

Unlike most runners, I've always enjoyed cross-training. Many people view it as a punishment for being injured or a way to burn a few extra calories on a running rest day. To me, cross-training is a good time to try something new or just take a mental break from the mileage grind. I incorporate all kinds of cross-training into my week even when I am training for a race—and as I've gotten older, the cross-training has kept me healthy and mostly injury-free.

One of my go-to forms of exercise is hands-free elliptical sessions. It's a nonimpact way to simulate running. It's almost like I'm getting the miles in without the pounding. Similarly, I enjoy going to the outdoor pool in the summertime to do deep-water running. I don't use a flotation device to do it. I just go to the deep end and

Cross-Training While Injured

Not all is lost when you're sidelined. You can still work on aerobic fitness, which will help ease the return to running after an injury. Concentrating on your cross-training schedule is also helpful in maintaining the lifestyle you love—and if you're still in that kind of routine, then it's likely you're staying upbeat, too, which is important in the healing process.

Here are a few cross-training tips for the injured runner.

1. Talk with your medical professional about what kinds of exercises are safe for you to do and when you can start doing them. Depending on what you're suffering from, some forms of cross-training can exacerbate the problem or prolong your recovery. It's important to have a full understanding of what you can do without causing additional harm.

2. Keep your heart rate up. It sounds simplistic, but runners are accustomed to naturally getting the cardiovascular benefits of exercise by putting one foot in front of the other. We tend to get lazy during other forms of exercise. So when you hop on the bike or elliptical, don't half-ass it. You want to feel like you're working

mimic my running stride, which can be a bit exaggerated in the water. The more quickly I move, the better I stay afloat. It's another good way to get many of the benefits of running without actually hitting the road.

Making sure I get in about two cross-training sessions per week has been critical to making it to 40 years of running. While running is about the only way to become a better runner (sorry, but there's no substitute for it), cross-training can help increase your cardio-

hard. Come up with an interval workout like you'd do in running to not only increase the benefits of your time on the machine, but also help the time pass quickly.

3. Choose your forms of cross-training carefully. Besides your doctor's advice (which is first and foremost), choose activities you enjoy doing or at least have been curious to try. If you hate to swim, then you're probably not going to do it. Find activities that are interesting and engaging to you.

4. Create structure. You have a distinct training plan when you're preparing for a race. When you're injured, you're preparing to return to running. Come up with a schedule like you would for your next marathon and stick to it in the same way.

5. Physical therapy comes first. If you have exercises and strength work you're supposed to perform or appointments at the Physical Therapy office, those come before anything else. So in a time crunch, if you're trying to decide whether to swim for an hour or do your PT exercises, those PT exercises have to take priority.

vascular fitness if you engage in forms of it that keep your heart rate up. It can also make you a more well-rounded athlete, which will lead to fewer injury risks. You get stronger by working different muscles, too.

I also recommend that new runners turn to cross-training while they're easing into a running routine. The extra days of exercise help improve fitness a little faster, which starts to make the running feel easier. This can help keep a newbie engaged and decrease the burnout (or frustration) factor. If somebody is trying to lose a few pounds, biking, swimming, or hitting the gym will also help achieve those goals.

For the injury-prone runner, substituting about 30 percent of weekly mileage with cross-training can help keep those problems at bay. Many of the country's top distance runners have used this method during times of trouble, when niggles start flaring up close to important competitions. In fact, Emily Infeld, the 2015 world championships bronze medalist in the 10,000 meters, had a stress fracture during the time she was building up to the 2016 Olympic Trials. Instead of wasting a lot of time worrying about her fitness, she got to work on a rigorous cross-training schedule. She only started running full-time again about 5 weeks before the trials, following 8 weeks of dedication to swimming, biking, and using the elliptical. She eased into running again cautiously and gradually, with plenty of reliance on the other fitness-building activities. The recipe led her to make her first Olympic team in the 10,000 meters in Rio de Janeiro.

NUTRITION

Talking about nutrition is akin to talking about politics or religion. Let it be known that I'm not prescribing a plan to anybody. I don't have a secret diet that has led me to all these years on my feet.

In fact, I hardly ever use the word *diet* because most people associate it with weight loss, which is not the goal. The goal is good health. I refer to it as a food regimen instead.

For years I have been a strict vegetarian. My reason is ethical—I have deep love for animals. So I haven't eaten meat for a very long while, and I practice veganism about 90 percent of the time (I sometimes think my recovery food of choice, pizza, is what prevents me from becoming a full vegan). Being vegan makes my adventures challenging at times, but I've picked up a few tips from some of the ultrarunners I follow, like Scott Jurek and Mike Wardian, who also travel the world on the run. Scott is vegan and Mike is vegetarian, and I'm in awe of how they're able to handle the globetrotting and the unfathomable mileage while adhering to their food regimen.

Mike, for example, ran seven marathons on seven continents in seven days at the beginning of 2017. He was worried about the availability of vegetarian fuel sources, which was going to play a huge part in his success. He was lucky enough to bring two bags of food along with him, including 20 packets of oatmeal, homemade granola, energy bars, almond butter, pretzel bread, ramen, and miso soup. He also packed some baby food to ensure that he had access to easily digestible fruits and vegetables in some of the far-flung locations like Antarctica.

No matter what your food philosophy is, three basic rules apply to runners.

1. Yes, you still need carbs. Turned to glycogen, they're the best and most efficient form of energy for endurance. You need carbohydrates to perform and recover. Just pick the right ones for the right times. If you're in the middle of a marathon, you need simple sugars like the kind that comes in gels and chews. If you're eating a meal, choose the more nutritious variety, which comes in the form of whole grains, fruits, and vegetables.

2. Eat within 30 minutes of a long run or hard effort. The window has become the stuff of running lore, but all the research backs it up. Eating about 250 calories of mostly carbs with a bit of protein will help get your recovery going faster.

3. Stay away from food wrapped in plastic. Your choices should be real and whole, not processed, chemical-laden food. A good rule of thumb is to shop the perimeter of the grocery store and stay away from the middle. Your meals and snacks should be comprised of quality food—lean protein, whole grains, legumes, fruits, vegetables, and healthy fats.

I don't like to overcomplicate my eating habits, but I can't help but think that sticking to mostly healthy choices and allowing myself indulgences from time to time has led to better running. What I believe is the bigger myth in the running community is that if "the furnace is hot enough anything will burn." It's simply not true. Better food leads to better athletic performance and a higher quality of life. Balance tends to be the critical factor in all things, including what we eat.

EMBRACING THE COMMUNITY

You can run all the miles, eat all the right foods, and lift all the weights you want. Sure, these strategies will make you a great athlete and enable a long career in running. But you won't find a bigger reason to stay in this sport than the people who are in it with you. I'm still here because of a community I can't imagine being without.

I have always held to the belief that's it's my job to encourage people to begin. I get them to their first race and I'll be the first to cheer them to the finish. But I've seen time and again that the running community will take it from there by welcoming all ages and abilities into its ranks. When I first began in the early 1980s, only the serious and the swift ran marathons. Now anybody can dream of finishing one—the access to coaches, training plans, clubs, and groups for recreational runners has exploded. Never have there been more resources and technology available to help anybody with a goal, whether it's to finish a 5K or win a 50 miler.

I go to these races—more than 40 of them a year—and I meet so many people who have overcome the most unfathomable odds to get there. People tell me how they have lost 150 pounds and are trying to break 3 hours in the marathon or that they're relieved to find a race on Sunday because the side effects of Friday's chemotherapy are harsher on Saturdays. It always gives me pause. I think of these people and these stories on the days that I wonder if my body can do it anymore. I want to be part of this world, and I don't care if I'm at the back of the pack, as long as I'm still having fun.

A big part of truly appreciating what we have in this sport is to make an effort to experience running from every angle and role you can. When you direct a race, for example, you'll never run another one without a great appreciation for the details that go into making it a success. As you look around you'll recognize the effort that went into securing the street permits, to soliciting finish line food donations, asking for sponsorships, and recruiting volunteers. You'll look at the race director and know how early she got up that morning to make sure the aid stations had enough water and the porta-potties were unlocked.

The day you decide to forgo a race to volunteer at it instead, you'll find out that helping others achieve their goals can be just as fulfilling as reaching your own. Maybe you'll stumble into a local running group and take a leadership role in its organization. There are many different ways to offer your time and skills—and the more generous you are with support, the more you'll get out of your running life.

As I near my retirement from *Runner's World,* I sometimes still can barely understand how a 10K in Moore Township, Pennsylvania, has brought me to this place. When George goaded me into it, he was urging me away from an inevitable dead end. At the time I didn't have a path forward or a compelling reason to improve upon a life that revolved around booze. I drove deliveries for a pharmaceutical company. Without a college degree, I had little direction—until I discovered where my running could eventually lead me, and the people it would bring into my life. Over all seven continents and points closer to home, it's no exaggeration to say that the act of putting one foot in front of the other changed my life completely. I've witnessed the power it has to transform so many others, too, and that's where I found my purpose: to inspire others to find health, joy, and meaning in running.

My first marathon had about 300 participants in it. Now a small 26.2-mile race is considered 5,000 people and New York City hosts 50,000 every November. When I started running, so few women lined up at races of any distance. Now they account for 57 percent of all race finishers in the United States. The doors are open for more people to participate than ever before, and they have flocked to be part of it for every reason imaginable.

But what I love most about racing remains consistent through the years. It allows us to dream, to realize the results of hard work, to challenge ourselves to take risks and be bold. For so many, just showing up at a starting line is an act of courage, a kind of bravery that teaches us how to push past our perceived limitations to find out if we can do—and be—something more.

Running has been at once an audacious adventure as well as a source of comfort and stability in my life. So, yes, I say race everything you can, for as long as you possibly can. And, again, never limit where your running can take you. I can't wait to see where it takes me next.

ACKNOWLEDGMENTS

BART

To all my colleagues at *Runner's World* and Rodale over the past 30 years. I worked with some amazing talent, and my coworkers have turned into friends for life. And to the Rodale family, thanks for the guidance, encouragement, and support over the past three decades. I have a debt of gratitude for what you have done for me.

ERIN

Much gratitude goes to Bart and Rodale Books for taking a chance on a first-time author; to my *Runner's World* colleagues, especially Scott Douglas and Sarah Lorge Butler, who provided advice, coffee, and mentorship; and to the Flagstaff, Arizona, running community, a family of friends who constantly remind me why this sport is always worth it.

INDEX

Boldface page references indicate photographs. Underscored references indicate boxed text or tables.

ABOUT THE AUTHORS

BART YASSO is chief running officer for *Runner's World* and one of the most beloved figures in the sport. Affectionately dubbed the "Mayor of Running," Bart is the public face of *Runner's World* at races in the United States and abroad. Bart has been with *Runner's World* since 1987, and has been instrumental in growing what was once a very small race sponsorship program to one that has linked the brand with thousands of races and millions of runners.

Bart is also known for creating Yasso 800s, a marathon-predictor workout that has been used by thousands of runners. His memoir, *My Life on the Run*, is a perennial top seller at the *Runner's World* booth (especially when Bart is on hand to sign copies!). He has also contributed to the *Runner's World Big Book of Marathon and Half Marathon Training* and *Runner's World Big Book of Running for Beginners*. One of the icons of the sport, Bart has been inducted into the Running USA Hall of Champions.

ERIN STROUT is a contributing editor at *Runner's World* and former senior editor at *Running Times*. Since 2013, she has covered the top levels of the sport, from the Boston Marathon to the Rio Olympics, for the *Runner's World* Newswire. As a freelance writer and editor with 20 years of journalism experience, Erin has also contributed to leading health and fitness publications and is a former staff reporter for the *Chronicle of Higher Education*. An avid runner, Erin lives in Flagstaff, Arizona.